Patients, Caregivers and Doctors

D1619068

Communication and Health Set

coordinated by
Laurence Corroy and Christelle Chauzal-Larguier

Volume 1

Patients, Caregivers and Doctors

Devices, Issues and Representations

Edited by

Laurence Corroy
Christelle Chauzal-Larguier

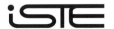

WILEY

First published 2023 in Great Britain and the United States by ISTE Ltd and John Wiley & Sons, Inc.

ISTE Ltd
27-37 St George's Road
London SW19 4EU
UK

www.iste.co.uk

John Wiley & Sons, Inc.
111 River Street
Hoboken, NJ 07030
USA

www.wiley.com

Any opinions, findings, and conclusions or recommendations expressed in this material are those of the author(s), contributor(s) or editor(s) and do not necessarily reflect the views of ISTE Group.

Library of Congress Control Number: 2023930936

British Library Cataloguing-in-Publication Data
A CIP record for this book is available from the British Library
ISBN 978-1-78630-893-1

Contents

Chapter 7. Taming Cancer. Affected Bodies, Mirrored Emotions and Challenges for Patients and Their Loved Ones   127
Anne VEGA and Ibtissem BEN DRIDI

Chapter 8. About Long Illnesses. Family Caregivers: Actors and Producers of Care and Health. The Case of Algeria   145
Aicha BENABED

Preface

Chronic and long-term illnesses, because of their lasting impact over time, expose the patient, the family caregiver[1] and the professional caregiver to multiple concerns that call into question the different systems implemented, the issues and the representations linked to them. The role of these three actors and the relationships that unite them can be questioned through the prism of a wide range of methods and processes, recent or not, implemented inside the care structures (recognition of peer helpers, recourse to cohesion techniques of care teams, telemedicine, proposal of new care offers, co-design of devices with the help of "collaborating" patients) as well as outside of them (homecare, distance learning, therapeutic education, assistance to family caregivers, digital devices, narrative medicine, "edutainment" within fictional television series, etc.).

P.1. Patients, caregivers and carers at the heart of a complex relational web

This book will study the patient, the carer and the caregiver according to their status and the care relationships that unite and

Preface written by Laurence CORROY and Christelle CHAUZAL-LARGUIER.
1 Article. L. 113-1-3 of the French Code of Social Action and Families (*Code de l'action sociale et des familles*): "Is considered as a close helper of an elderly person, their spouse, the partner with whom the person has concluded a civil solidarity pact or their cohabitant, a parent or an ally, defined as close helpers, […], who helps them, regularly and frequently, on a non-professional basis, to accomplish all or part of the acts or activities of daily life".

divide them. Today, patients, carers and caregivers are subject to a burdensome, anxiety-provoking climate, marked by a feeling of insecurity, whether material, professional or emotional, prompting them to engage in introspection that can lead to a reconsideration of their own role.

The patient is led to reflect, in particular, on their ability to maintain a positive attitude when their bruised body causes pain and questions and when the professional, social and economic environment is disrupted (Lefort and Psiuk 2019). The caregiver, trained in a form of providing medicine designed to relieve the ills of the body, rather than moral suffering, works in a tense professional context, generated by a health system on the verge of implosion (lack of staff, difficult working conditions, unattractive salaries). The degraded care sacrifices the human dimension, inflicting on the caregiver a feeling of helplessness, a loss of professional ideal (Delieutraz 2012) and a heavy emotional burden (Chahraoui et al. 2011; Petiau 2016). The latter leads to question the limits of the traditional approach of "caring" centered on the acts themselves, increasingly convinced that "care taking", centered on the person receiving care, should be adopted instead (Hesbeen 2012). The family caregiver, little or poorly prepared (Leduc et al. 2013), prey to strong emotions (Mallon and Le Bihan-Youinou. 2017), questions their ability to reconcile their caregiving activities with professional and personal activities (Le Bihan-Youinou and Martin 2006; Fontaine 2009). An unrecognized shadow actor (Bloch 2012), they have difficulty thinking of themselves and accepting themselves as such (Bricka 2016).

Even though the knowledge and skills of the caregiver are recognized as scientific expertise, "no one today can dispute the importance of the relational attitude in care activities" (Formarier 2007, p. 33). Since patients are not satisfied with being passive (Pierron 2007) and families do not accept being left out, they all demand greater involvement in care protocols. While the dyad between the patient and the caregiver appears to be of little relevance, institutional, medical and lay discourses evoke the importance of a third category of actors, the close caregivers[2] whose important role in

---

2 The number of family caregivers continues to grow and now reaches 11 million people ("Aidants: le temps des solutions?", *Ipsos/Macif survey*, 2020).

the care pathway is widely recognized even though the abundant literature on the subject testifies to the gray areas (Buthion and Godé 2014). The tripartite relational dimension in care is unavoidable. Patients, caregivers and carers have never so much sought, or even demanded, a more human approach to care relationships while the caregiver experiences difficulties in being able to invest in it. This triad of actors, which is part of the long term, must deal with long treatments for which the territories of understanding and the horizons of expectation of each require adjustments (Sicard 2002; Kentish-Barnes 2010; Maupetit and Fondras 2011), dialogue and assistance. Without this, the feeling of solitude felt individually by the different parties can increase (Canouï and Mauranges 1998) and cause them to sink into exhaustion, especially since the caregiver, for example, does not dare ask for help (Coudin and Gely-Nargeot 2003).

How can the relational quality of care be reconciled with a context of increased tension for the caregiver? How are the patients' relationships with doctors staged when healing medicine shows its limits? What is the place and role of the caregiver when holistic medicine, which aims to treat the person in a global way, is struggling to be developed within the hospital environment? How sustainable is the patient–caregiver–caregiver relationship model (Mitnick et al. 2010) in the event of the failure of one or more of the actors involved? Is the support of other actors (associations, private organizations, individuals, public structures and institutions) conceivable if not possible and how is it represented? These are the questions that the relationships between patients, caregivers and carers and the roles of each can raise. To answer these questions, it is essential to reflect on the representations of each person.

P.2. Representations of patients, carers and caregivers in discourse

The aim of this book is also to fill a gap in qualitative research on these issues when, as Rul and Carnevale (2014, p. 241) note, they "allow for the generation of knowledge about social processes or behaviors, or the experiences of people confronted with a situation in a given context". While traditionally, the denomination of the patient[3] refers the patient to their condition of being consumed by suffering and devoid of knowledge, digital platforms have increased this information (Cases 2017) and the legislation[4] has recognized their right in this regard, shaking up the notion of an asymmetrical relationship between patient and caregiver. The patient has become a "knowing being" for want of a "savant" (Le Pen 2009, p. 260), an actor of their own health as envisaged by research on patient "empowerment" (Hibbard et al. 2004).

The importance of the relational dimension of care and the problems of representations raise questions about the feelings and affects that arise in the different actors (patients, caregivers, carers) in relation to chronic diseases. This requires a reflection on the researcher's methodological approaches to study these dimensions. Phenomenological interpretive analysis allows us to discover and study in depth the experience of illness and the care process. It is increasingly used in psychological research, particularly in health and clinical psychology (Antoine and Smith 2017). The linguistic analysis of discourse, which is still underdeveloped in this field of research (Garric and Herbland 2020), allows the researcher to let these actors express themselves and recount their experiences. Speech is then a key resource that must be studied for its own sake (Rossi 2011) because it is the means of accessing a "contextualization" of the individual and/or collective experience. In this field of research, playful approaches through games can also allow actors to distance themselves from the situations of suffering experienced, both in the context of care activities and in the experience of illness, while allowing the researcher to give a participatory dimension to the studies.

---

3 Patient refers to the Latin "*pati*" literally meaning "one who suffers".

4 Article L. 1111-2 of the French Health Code, which came into force on October 1st, 2020: "Everyone has the right to be informed about their state of health. This information concerns the different investigations, treatments or preventive actions that are proposed, their usefulness, their possible urgency, their consequences, the frequent or serious risks normally foreseeable that they entail, as well as the other possible solutions and the foreseeable consequences in the event of refusal".

The importance of the communication and information media where this discourse can be collected must also be discussed. Digital platforms allow patients to talk about their symptoms and treatments, to discuss their care pathways and their relationship with their doctors and the care team. Websites (Kinnane and Milne 2010; Dolce 2011) and forums dedicated to caregivers, with their vocation of mutual aid and exchange of advice, and also by the information and training offered, tend to break their isolation, to bring comfort (Dubreuil and Hazif-Thomas 2013) while remaining compatible with their daily lives (Nabarette 2002). Finally, testimonies can be a tool to mediate the "denial of recognition" (Charlier 2018) that one or more actors in the above-mentioned triangular relationship is/are confronted with, or to publicize the changes that have occurred, particularly in life courses (disorganization and reorganization of family ties, for example) (Dupré La Tour and Gorlero 2012; Bonnet-Llompart and Laurent 2020).

On another note, work on television series has already shown the importance in the spectatorial experience of television series and edutainment related to health (Singhal et al. 2004; Barthes 2016), whether it be prevention or apprehension of certain diseases.

Far from being anecdotal, these testimonies and stories are part of what can be defined as narrative medicine (Charon 2015; Goupy and Lejeunne 2016), which tends to develop competence and increased vigilance on the part of the patient (in the relationship they have with their own body and restores them as actors in their lives and potentially in their recovery) and of the caregiver (in the relationship that binds them to the sick loved one and repositioning them as an actor independent of the person being cared for).

Putting into words the ills experienced, distanced by language and lived experiences, far from constituting a unified whole, can also question in return the role of medical teams, the ambivalences felt, and constitute for the carers a reflexive spur on their practices while providing them with an extremely rich documentation of a multiplicity of cases. Indeed, as Dagognet (2009: 172) points out, "medicine is hermeneutics, a science of interpreting what is in front of our eyes and what we cannot see" and for which the discourses and verbal exchanges constitute indispensable methodological tools.

This book questions the devices, the stakes and the representations related to chronic and long-term illnesses by questioning the way patients define themselves, the relationships they establish with their caregivers and how the figure of the caregiver can be staged as a necessary adjuvant to the patient, whether it be testimonies on digital platforms or in fictional universes, and also in everyday life, within organizational structures (medical structures, companies, associations) and private structures (private environment of the patient and the caregiver). In order to provide elements of reflection and answers to these questions, teacher-researchers and professionals from various fields of research and competences belonging to two disciplines have collaborated in this book: information and communication sciences through the analysis of the representations of patients, care staff and carers through communication media, discourses, arguments and rhetorical figures mobilized; management sciences by studying the organizational and communicational devices of public and private companies with these targets.

To answer these questions, this book presents research conducted around two closely complementary themes. The first part of the book highlights the challenges and opportunities of digital and playful devices for patients, caregivers and carers. Julie Pavillet and Aurélie Dumas are interested in a game-based device for occupational health prevention. Using a collaborative and participatory methodology, the nursing staff of a long-term geriatric care unit at the Grenoble Alpes University Hospital were asked to discuss their work in order to express their emotions and affects without violence. Through the affective and relational dynamics that the Dixit® card game creates, a team in pain manages, through individual and collective reflection on professional practices, to acquire new resources intended to facilitate the establishment of work groups that can lead to organizational changes within the hospital.

Nathalie Garric and Frédéric Pugnière-Saavedra use a situated analysis in discourse analysis combining a quantitative textometric approach and a qualitative enunciative approach to show that certain digital devices, in this case the blogs of which they are the authors, give caregivers the opportunity to provide a discourse other than the existing institutional discourse on their subject, which escapes certain normative constraints on the experience of caregiving as it is presented in media and legal discourses. Confronting this digital corpus with a corpus of individual interviews of caregivers and families, the authors conclude that this discourse does not play the role of a counter-discourse because it is constructed in and for a restricted community of people with the aim of constructing themselves and defining their role.

Ambre Davat and Fabienne Martin-Juchat detail the methodology, justify the interest and address the ethical and societal issues of the co-design project. With a group of patients, the aim was to co-design a study enabling the development of information and communication devices for future patients with chronic heart failure and equipped with connected implants. The chosen method was based on interviews allowing the collection of the experiences of the "collaborating" patients through their stories of affects related to their care path. The patients' role was to participate in the definition of the major questioning areas of the study, to validate the hypotheses and the test method chosen. This work led to the collective and organizational dynamics involved in the follow-up of this chronic disease emerging.

Emna Cherif and Corinne Rochette look at the opportunities and challenges of highlighting healthcare offers on the websites of health institutions. This is a response to the impossibility for these organizations to communicate as commercial enterprises, to an exacerbated competition between hospital structures and to an evolution of patients' expectations. The study of 17 institutional communication websites of hospitals (university hospitals, clinics and cancer centers) allows us to assess their patient orientation. Are patient-centric markers identifiable? How are they expressed? Being patient-centric is not present in a similar way in all the sites studied, through more or less extensive information processes and the implementation of specific resources and skills, thus highlighting cultural and behavioral approaches to this orientation.

Alexis Meyer and Christelle Chauzal-Larguier question the online marketing communication strategy pursued by seven French thermal spa establishments and one thalassotherapy center offering a mini-cure for caregivers and analyze the discourse held, in particular by using comparative analysis. Two complementary methods are mobilized: a study of the dedicated pages of the websites of these establishments and the content analysis of in-depth interviews with actors of the spa sector. Can't the purely informative discourse evolve or even deviate towards a real commercial communication to promote some services? The caregiver then becomes not only an informative but also a commercial target. The offer so proposed constitutes a strong stake for thermalism and contributes to its repositioning.

The second part focuses more closely on the narrative and hermeneutic medicine of the patient and caregiver.

Laurence Corroy and Emilie Roche explore how the French series *Demain nous appartient*, broadcast daily by TF1 since 2017, Monday through Friday, dramatizes how a recurring character on the show faces breast cancer and how loved ones react. This ensemble show and family series offers locations that are easily identified by fans of the series: high school, police station, hospital, etc. Patients, caregivers and doctors are at the heart of hospital plots that allow, through the narrative construction of the series, the feature of several different points of view and protagonists who evolve according to the twists and turns of a specific narrative arc. The one analyzed by the two researchers corresponds to two months of broadcasting, during which the director of the hospital's general medicine department becomes a patient with breast cancer. During this situation of personal crisis, the narrative medicine of the doctor turned patient, who evokes doubts and fears, while having expert knowledge and a supportive professional and intimate entourage, being herself of the party, intertwine. However, despite the fact that the character is familiar with the world of care, she nevertheless feels shock at the diagnosis.

From the triad of doctor to patient, carer and caregiver, preventive discourses and norms are disseminated, placing the series at the heart of a device considered to be edutainment: fans of *Demain nous appartient*, whose emotional attachment to the series and to the recurring characters is strong, receive, over the course of the episodes, preventive messages and models of valued or criticized behaviors (good care vs. bad care, the importance of screening, rapid care of patients, etc.) which emerge in the background.

Leaving the world of fiction, Anne Vega and Ibtissem Ben Dridi shed light on the way in which relatives are progressively led to take charge of and support their family members suffering from cancer. The announcement of the disease is experienced as a trauma, a shockwave that must be gradually absorbed – the help of family members is therefore crucial. In addition to psychological difficulties, patients may also be in a precarious financial and family situation. While patients from well-to-do or even very well-to-do social categories may feel more at ease with the medical profession and are better able to discuss and negotiate treatment protocols, those from working-class backgrounds are more apprehensive about making their point of view heard. The two authors show to what extent, in this case, the help of relatives, extended to colleagues, neighbors and other patients encountered who form a supportive entourage, can be decisive. A diversified support network allows patients to acquire empowerment with regard to their illness and also with regard to the medical profession, partially freeing them from the asymmetrical positions between "knowers" and patients and from injunctions that may be impossible to follow to the latter. The caregiver can also, in socially disadvantaged family contexts, develop skills similar to those of a home care worker.

The field study conducted by Aicha Benabed in the Algerian context shows how caregivers are led to develop the medical know-how which is extremely important for the very longevity of the patient they care for. This "medical work" (Strauss 1992) is illustrated by the family trajectories that the researcher was able to identify and present. The testimonies demonstrate the scope and diversity of the tasks performed. Learning to assess the weak signs of the disease in order to evaluate the condition of the sick family member and understand their symptoms makes it possible to anticipate their daily needs. This watchfulness places the caregiver in a state of extreme vigilance, which proves to be exhausting in the long run and a source of anxiety. Help does not only develop in the family context; the caregivers interviewed show that when their loved ones were hospitalized, their care work continued, as hospitals are understaffed. It is the women on whom all care work rests. The author thus notes a gendered and asymmetrical division of care in the Algerian context, which weighs heavily on female caregivers, whose well-being is undermined.

Managing emotions, ambivalent feelings and even guilt can be difficult and even painful for caregivers. If caregivers develop hermeneutics of the patient they are caring for, hermeneutics of the self is just as fundamental. Digital platforms, allowing relative anonymity and a wider circulation of caregivers' dilemmas and difficulties, often appear to be an easy way to speak out and testify. However, is the platformization of relationships and communications without impact on the type of discourse delivered and the emotions expressed? Abdelhadi Bellachhab, Olga Galatanu and Valérie Rochaix provide enlightening answers by comparing two communicational devices and two corpora – the first corresponding to 10 discussions from a digital platform where caregivers of Alzheimer's patients express themselves and the second to 10 semi-directive biographical interviews conducted as part of a scientific project. The results show that the modalities of emotional expression, as well as the emotions themselves, depend on the communication devices observed. If guilt, for example, is experienced and discussed on the online discussion forum, it hardly appears during the discussions conducted with the researchers. It seems, therefore, that addressing peers who share common experiential experiences on a digital platform is viewed quite differently compared to testifying with researchers. It would be hasty to conclude, however, that emotions are not expressed in front of scientists, some of them are on the contrary strongly evoked, notably the caregivers' constant fear of doing wrong.

The difficulty of taking care of someone who gives their time, love and energy to a close family member, finally led the DanaeCare team to propose a co-construction of a territory that facilitates assistance. André Simonnet, Julia Gudefin and Maya Chabane indeed emphasize a problem often underestimated by caregivers concerning the impact of territorial networking on their daily life. The fact that the public authorities have thought of care as primarily intended for the elderly and the loss of autonomy is not without consequences. However, assistance is diverse, transgenerational and concerns multiple pathologies. They do not fit easily into the categories conceived by public policies. The project led by the authors, DanaeCare, is therefore part of a territorial logic, that of the department of Saint-Étienne and adopts a concerted approach. In the tripartite relationship between caregiver, carer and patient, it is important that each actor be recognized, especially the carers who ensure a crucial coordination for the patient. The lengthening of patients' lives, and hence the chronicity of illnesses and treatments, are profoundly transforming this tripartite relationship, where the patient can gradually become an expert on their illness and the caregiver a fine interpreter of the loved one to whom they provide support, while developing multiple skills. The DanaeCare project highlights the importance of co-constructing adapted solutions within a given territory.

The experiences and disciplines brought together in this book shed light on the complexity and interest of paying close attention to the relationships that develop between patients, care staff and family members. The dualities between those who know and those who do not seem less and less operational. Thinking about the actors in interaction, respecting the patient's word as well as the caregiver's role in order to provide the most appropriate solutions will undoubtedly improve the quality of care, and also the care relationships.

February 2023

P.3. References

Antoine, P. and Smith, J.A. (2017). Saisir l'expérience : présentation de l'analyse phénoménologique interprétative comme méthodologie qualitative en psychologie. *Psychologie française*, 62(4), 373–385.

Barthes, S. (2016). Panique à la télé : la résistance bactérienne vue par les séries. *Questions de communication*, 29, 111–134.

Bloch, M.-A. (2012). Les aidants et l'émergence d'un nouveau champ de recherche Interdisciplinaire. *Vie sociale*, 4(4), 11–29.

Bonnet-Llompart, M. and Laurent, A. (2020). Désorganisation des liens familiaux et réactivation des conflits chez les aidants confrontés à la maladie... d'Alzheimer de leur mère. *Dialogue*, 3(229), 123–141.

Bricka, B. (2016). *Des vies (presque) ordinaires, Paroles d'aidants*. Éditions de l'Atelier, Paris.

Buthion, V. and Godé, C. (2014). Les proches-aidants, quels rôles dans la coordination du parcours de soins des personnes malades. *Journal de gestion et d'économie médicales*, 32(37), 501–519.

Canouï, P. and Mauranges, A. (1998). *Le syndrome d'épuisement professionnel des soignants*. Masson, Paris.

Cases, A.-S. (2017). L'e-santé : l'empowerment du patient connecté. *Journal de gestion et d'économie médicales*, 35(4), 137–158.

Chahraoui, K., Bioy, A., Cras, E., Gilles, F., Laurent, A., Valache, B., Quenot, J.-P. (2011). Vécu psychologique des soignants en réanimation : une étude exploratoire et qualitative. *Annales françaises d'anesthésie et de réanimation*, 242–248.

Charlier, E. (2018). Aidants proches : une reconnaissance en demi-teinte? *La Revue nouvelle*, 4(4), 59–64.

Charon, R. (2015). *Médecine narrative, rendre hommage aux histoires de maladies*. Sipayat, Paris.

Coudin, G. and Gely-Nargeot, M.C. (2003). Le paradoxe de l'aide aux aidants ou la réticence des aidants informels à recourir aux services. *Neurologie – Psychiatrie – Gériatrie*, 3, 19–23.

Dagognet, F. (2009). L'imagerie médicale, une ambivalence certaine, quoique relative. *Recherches en psychanalyse*, 2(8), 170–174.

Delieutraz, S. (2012). Le vécu d'impuissance chez le soignant : entre pertes et élan retrouvé. *Cliniques*, 2(4), 146–162.

Dolce, M.C. (2011). The internet as a source of health information: Experiences of cancer survivors and caregivers with healthcare providers. *Oncology Nursing Forum*, 38, 353–359.

Dubreuil, A. and Hazif-Thomas, C. (2013). Les aidants et la santé sur internet ou les "aidantnautes" s'entraident. *Neurologie/Psychiatrie/Gériatrie*, 13, 250–255.

Dupré La Tour, M. and Gorlero, C. (2012). Quand la maladie révèle et réveille les souffrances familiales. *Dialogue*, 3(197), 57–68.

Fontaine, R. (2009). Aider un parent âgé se fait-il au détriment de l'emploi ? *Retraite et Société*, 2(58), 31–61.

Formarier, M. (2007). La relation de soin, concepts et finalités. *Recherche en soins infirmiers*, 2(89), 33–42.

Garric, N. and Herbland, A. (2020). Présentation. Nouveaux discours de la santé et soin relationnel. *Langage et société*, 1(169), 15–30.

Goupy, F. and Lejeunne, C. (eds) (2016). *La médecine narrative, une révolution pédagogique ?* Édition Med Line, Paris.

Hesbeen, W. (2012). *Penser le soin en réadaptation. Agir pour le devenir de la personne*. Seli Arslan, Paris.

Hibbard, J., Stockard, J., Mahoney, E., Tusler, M. (2004). Development of the patient activation measure (PAM): Conceptualizing and measuring activation in patients and consumers. *Health Services Research*, 39(4), 1005–1026.

Kentish-Barnes, N. (2010). Vécu de la parole en réanimation : complexités et ambiguïtés de la relation soignants-soignés/famille. In *La philosophie du soin. Éthique, médecine et société*, Benaroyo, L., Lefève, C., Mino, J.-C., Worms, F. (eds). Presses Universitaires de France, Paris.

Kinnane, N.A. and Milne, D.J. (2010). The role of the internet in supporting and informing carers of people with cancer: A literature review. *Supportive Care in Cancer*, 18(9), 1123–1136.

Le Bihan-Youinou, B. and Martin, C. (2006). Travailler et prendre soin d'un parent âgé dépendant. *Revue Travail, genre et sociétés*, 16(2), 77–96.

Le Pen, C. (2009). "Patient" ou "personne malade" ? *Revue économique*, 60(2), 257–272.

Leduc, F., Jung, E., Lozac'h, C. (2013). Former les aidants : comment ? Pourquoi ? Pour quoi faire ? *Gérontologie et société*, 36(47), 189–198.

Lefort, H. and Psiuk, T. (2019). *Patient partenaire, patient expert*. Vuibert, Paris.

Mallon, I. and Le Bihan-Youinou, B. (2017). Le poids des émotions : une réflexion sur les variations de l'intensité de l'(entr)aide familiale auprès des proches dépendants. *Sociologie*, 8(2), 121–138.

Maupetit, C. and Fondras, M. (2011). Patient, famille, soignant : un vécu commun, une (in)compréhension réciproque. *Médecine palliative*, 10(4), 173–177.

Mitnick, S., Leffler, C., Hood, V. (2010). Family caregivers, patients and physicians: Ethical guidance to optimize relationships. *Journal of General Internal Medicine*, 25(3), 255–260.

Nabarette, H. (2002). L'internet médical et la consommation d'information par les patients. *Réseaux*, 4(114), 249–286.

Petiau, A. (2016). Ne dites surtout pas que vous êtes médecin : plaidoyer pour une prise en compte du vécu des soignants. *Cahiers critiques de thérapie familiale et de pratiques de réseaux*, 2(57), 103–118.

Pierron, J.-P. (2007). Une nouvelle figure du patient ? Les transformations contemporaines de la relation de soins. *Sciences sociales et santé*, 25(2), 43–66.

Rossi, I. (2011). La parole comme soin : cancer et pluralisme thérapeutique. *Anthropologie & Santé*, 2 [Online]. Available at: http://journals.openedition.org.ezproxy.uca.fr/anthropologiesante/659.

Rul, B. and Carnevale, F. (2014). Recherche en soins palliatifs : intérêt des méthodes qualitatives. *Médecine Palliative*, 13(5), 241–248.

Sicard, D. (2002). Le patient et le médecin. In *Que ferons-nous de l'homme ? Biologie, médecine et société*, Semaines sociales de France (ed.). Paris, Bayard.

Singhal, A., Cody, M., Rogers, E.M., Sabido, M. (eds) (2004). *Entertainment-Education and Social Change. History, Research and Practices*. L. Erlbaum, Mahwah.

Strauss, A. (1992). *La Trame de la négociation* (reprinted by Baszanger, I.). L'Harmattan, Paris.

Author Biographies

Abdelhadi BELLACHHAB

Abdelhadi Bellachhab has a PhD in linguistics from the Université de Nantes. He is a member of the PREFics laboratory (EA4246). Located at the interface of semantics and pragmatics, his research focuses on the construction of meaning and the discursive construction of identities (health, didactics, institutional discourse), the acquisition of semantic and pragmatic skills, contrastive and intercultural pragmatics and conceptual semantics.

Ibtissem BEN DRIDI

Ibtissem Ben Dridi is an anthropologist and research engineer at the *École des Hautes Études en Santé Publique* (EHESP) and a researcher affiliated with the Arènes laboratory (UMR CNRS 6051). She has been involved in the CORSAC project (Coordination of ambulatory care during the acute therapeutic phase of cancer) since 2011 and in the CANOPÉE project (Cancers in people followed for severe psychological disorders) since 2020.

Aicha BENABED

Aicha Benabed is a lecturer in sociology and anthropology at the Université d'Oran 2 (Algeria) and a researcher associated with the research unit in social sciences and health (GRAS). Her research areas are: health (family, reproductive health and infertility), ART and kinship. She is currently working on care, gender relations and health.

Maya CHABANE

Maya Chabane holds a bachelor's degree in Sociology and a master's degree in Social Policies and Territorial Development from the Université Jean Monnet de Saint-Étienne. Her research paper, entitled *"Valorisation du rôle et du statut des proches-aidants"*, includes a sociological analysis of the place of family caregivers in the healthcare system and society. The ecology of caregiver–patient–caregiver relationships is thus a relevant entry point for the analysis of the organization of healthcare. She is currently in charge of the DanaeCare association and coordinates the Escale des Aidants project in the Loire region.

Christelle CHAUZAL-LARGUIER

Christelle Chauzal-Larguier is a lecturer in Management Sciences at the Université Clermont Auvergne and a member of the Communication and Societies Laboratory (EA 4647). Her research work focuses on corporate communication and the themes of corporate social responsibility and solidarity policy within the company (Christelle Chauzal-Larguier and Sébastien Rouquette, *La solidarité, une affaire d'entreprise ?* Presses universitaires Blaise Pascal 2018). This last theme is studied through the employees who are caregivers and the devices imagined to help them.

Emna CHERIF

Emna Cherif is a lecturer in Management Sciences at the IAE, Université Clermont Auvergne and a member of CleRMA (Clermont Recherche Management – EA 3849). She is in charge of the Marketing–Sales specialization and her research focuses on digital marketing, the adoption of new technologies and the digitalization of healthcare.

Laurence CORROY

Laurence Corroy is a university professor of Information and Communication Sciences at the *Centre de recherche sur les médiations* (CREM – EA 3476) at the Université de Lorraine. Her work is structured around two main areas of research: critical education in media, digital and information literacy, and the communicative practices of young people; and health education, in particular through the creation of health issues in the public space, television dramas and related media discourses and representations.

Her latest published works are as follows:

– Corroy, L. and Raichvarg, D (eds) (2020). "Génération(s) santé" dossier. *Revue française des sciences de l'information et de la communication*, 19.

– Corroy, L. and Ricaud, P. (2019). *Utopies et médias de masse*. ISTE Éditions, Paris, London.

– Corroy, L. (2016). *Education et médias, la créativité à l'ère du numérique*. ISTE Éditions, Paris, London.

– Université de Lorraine – CREM.

Ambre DAVAT

Ambre Davat is a postdoctoral researcher at the Université Grenoble Alpes. After studying engineering, she specialized in the study of speech and completed her thesis in social robotics. Her research focuses on the socio-affective issues related to the use of new digital technologies in everyday life.

TIMC/Gresec/IPhiG.

Aurélia DUMAS

Aurélia Dumas is a lecturer in Information and Communication Sciences at the Communication and Societies Laboratory (EA 4647) of the Université Clermont Auvergne (UCA). Her research is in the field of organizational communication and focuses on occupational health and the prevention measures implemented within organizations.

Olga GALATANU

Olga Galatanu has a PhD and is qualified to direct research in language sciences. She is also DHC in science and philosophy at the University of Turku. She is an emeritus professor at the Université de Nantes and a member of the PREFics laboratory (EA 4246). Her research, at the semantic–pragmatic interface, focuses on the generation and reconstruction of linguistic meaning and the discursive construction of the self and the world. This research has led her to develop a theory of linguistic meaning, the semantics of argumentative possibilities. She is the author of three monographs and co-author of 10 collective works.

Nathalie GARRIC

Nathalie Garric is a professor at the Université de Nantes where she teaches pragmatics, enunciation and discourse analysis. She conducts her research at the PREFics laboratory (EA 4246) of the UBS (Université Bretagne-Sud). Her analyses focus on the study of contemporary social issues that occupy the public debate, with a particular interest in issues involving vulnerable actors. Her research is based on French discourse analysis, combining qualitative indexical analysis and quantitative textometric analysis in a complementary way, with an applicative perspective.

Julia GUDEFIN

Julia Gudefin is a doctor of law specializing in environmental law. She spent the first years of her professional life in teaching and research at the Université Jean Moulin Lyon 3 and carrying out teaching missions in Armenia and Egypt. The ecosystemic vision necessary to protect the environment has, as a patient, led her to see the health sector as an ecosystem rich in actors and interconnections within the medical environment in which they evolve and which must be preserved. She is also the co-founder and co-director of the DanaeCare association.

Fabienne MARTIN-JUCHAT

Fabienne Martin-Juchat is currently a university professor in Information and Communication Sciences at the Université Grenoble Alpes. She is developing an anthropology of bodily and affective communication, mediated or not by technologies. She is a member of the GRESEC Laboratory and is responsible for a research program on the place of the body and emotions in the construction of collective action and in organizational communication. She develops research partnerships based on participatory methodologies. She relies on narratives of affect to understand organizational logics and the relationships between actors and devices.

Alexis MEYER

Director of the Office de Tourisme et du Thermalisme de Bourbon-Lancy, Alexis Meyer is a lecturer at the Université Clermont Auvergne. After studying Strategic Information and Market Action with an international focus, he first worked in the marketing department of a mass retail group in Lyon, then became the director of a spa resort tourist office and specialized in new marketing strategies applied to tourism and spa services. For the past six years, he has been teaching business and marketing subjects at the IUT Clermont Auvergne.

Julie PAVILLET

Julie Pavillet is a work and organizational psychologist, and a professional risk prevention specialist attached to the Grenoble Alpes University Hospital (CHUGA) Workplace Health Team. She is the initiator of various prevention approaches (ORSOSA), which focus on improving quality of life and working conditions. She carries out actions with hospital staff, in particular by proposing collective support with a view to preserving health at work.

Frédéric PUGNIÈRE-SAAVEDRA

Frédéric Pugnière-Saavedra is a lecturer in linguistics at the Université Bretagne Sud (UBS) and carries out his research activities within the PREFics-Ubs (EA 4246). His work focuses on discourse analysis as a central disciplinary approach to apprehend syntax and lexicon in the construction of meaning, mainly through corpora relating to the field of social space: procedures for reporting children in danger, interviews with sex offenders, interviews with the homeless, procedures and discourse on the demolition of large housing estates, archives of chats from the association fighting against suicide, and interviews with caregivers of Alzheimer's patients.

Valérie ROCHAIX

Valérie Rochaix is a lecturer in linguistics at the Université de Tours and a member of the LLL (UMR-CNRS 7270). Her work in semantics, pragmatics and discourse analysis focuses on institutional and health discourses. She is a member of the ACCMADIAL project (IRESP, 2020–2022).

– Garric, N., Pugnière-Saavedra, F., Rochaix, V., *Construction langagière de la figure de l'aidant du malade d'Alzheimer : dénominations et mise en mots interdiscursive dans les pratiques.* CORELA – COgnition, REprésentation, LAngage, CERLICO – Cercle Linguistique du Centre et de l'Ouest (France), 2020 (hal-02899867).

Emilie ROCHE

Emilie Roche is a lecturer in Information and Communication Sciences at the Université Sorbonne Nouvelle and a media historian. A specialist in media representations, particularly of armed conflicts and violence (Roche 2008), she has worked on the Algerian War, conflicts related to decolonization and terrorism (Roche 2017, 2018). Within the research center on social links (CERLIS), she works on media representations of health (Corroy and Roche 2016). Since 2009, she has co-led a seminar on the magazine press as a source and object of history at the Centre d'histoire de Sciences Po (CHSP) and later at the Laboratoire Communication et Politique (LCP) (Roche et al. 2018).

Corinne ROCHETTE

Corinne Rochette is a university professor at the IAE Clermont Auvergne and a member of CleRMA (Clermont Recherche Management, EA 3849). She created a master's degree in public management and then in management of medico-social and health organizations. She is co-founder and holder of the research chair in health and territories of the Clermont Auvergne University Foundation. She is a member of the board of the International Association of Public Management Research and an expert for several public organizations. She studies the transformations of public organizations and services. Part of her work focuses on the health sector with the study of access to care, innovative organizational arrangements, governance and patient pathways. She currently directs six theses. Her work has resulted in about 100 academic contributions (articles and conferences).

Université Clermont Auvergne – CleRMa.

André SIMONNET

André Simonnet is a photojournalist and documentary filmmaker. What is fascinating about this profession is the opportunity to enter the backstage of our societies and to build a reflection fed by the testimonies of the actors on the ground, decision-makers and academic actors. But it is as a chronic patient affected by frequent aura migraines that he began studying hospitals and was able to experience a wide variety of relationships with caregivers. It seemed important to him to understand why there were such great relational differences from one caregiver to the next and what impacts the caregiver had on their daily professional and personal lives. Starting from a finding based on a relationship between two people (caregiver/patient), the reflection naturally extended to the environment in which this relationship evolves and the issues that this implies for caregivers, patients, caregivers and health systems.

He is also the co-founder and co-director of DanaeCare.

Anne VEGA

Anne Vega is a socio-anthropologist and researcher at the Université de Nanterre, affiliated with the SOPHIAPOL laboratory. She is an HSS expert for the INCA (French National Cancer Institute) and the ANSM (French National Agency for the Safety of Medicines and Health Products). Since 2011, she has been coordinating the CORSAC research project (Coordination of ambulatory care during the acute therapeutic phase of cancer).

PART 1

Stakes and Opportunities of Digital and Playful Devices for Patients, Caregivers and Care Providers

1

The Use of Games as an Innovative Prevention Method for Discussing Work with Hospital Healthcare Staff

This study is based on the results of an exploratory investigation conducted with caregivers of a long-term care unit. Through the implementation of an innovative prevention method, thanks to the resources of the game, the objective was to recreate a collective work within suffering care units. Through the back door of the game, this is about facilitating the particularly affective expression of caregivers in order to rebuild the bonds between staff members, encouraging the discussion about the work within the collectives. The game can mediate an individual and collective reflection on professional practices in order to provide caregivers with new resources useful for the (re-)creation of work collectives, sources of organizational changes within the hospital institution.

1.1. Introduction

This study is based on the results of a field experiment conducted with caregivers at the Grenoble Alpes University Hospital (*Centre hospitalier universitaire Grenoble Alpes*, CHUGA) caring for elderly polypathological patients. It follows a previous research study (Dumas

Chapter written by Julie PAVILLET and Aurélia DUMAS.

and Pavillet 2018) within the framework of a research program[1] concerning the question of the place and role of emotions within the hospital institution and more specifically among health managers. As an extension of this research, which was conducted using a partnership approach that brought together both social science researchers and professionals from the university hospital and which led to several publications (Dujardin and Lépine 2018; Lépine and Martin-Juchat 2018; Martin-Juchat et al. 2018a, 2018b), we felt it would be interesting to continue our exploration of the field and to further develop the question of how to take affects into account in the support of healthcare personnel. The results of this previous empirical research conducted with healthcare managers have shown how the mastery of affects is similar to emotional skills expected of healthcare staff by the hospital institution but constitutes a task carried out individually, invisible and unrecognized. Although healthcare personnel are strongly solicited from the point of view of the emotional burden claimed in their daily work, and even though this problem is widely known[2], individualizing logics persist, leading to a non-recognition and non-management of the affects at work within the hospital institution.

Based on this observation, we proposed to continue our field experimentation using a partnership approach mobilizing a so-called participatory methodology (Lépine and Martin-Juchat 2020). We wondered about the possibilities of rebuilding bonds of trust between staff members through the implementation of an innovative prevention method within the hospital institution, using games. Through the game, the aim was to approach the organization and team dynamics differently by introducing a "new object" that would make it possible to decentralize the work problem in order to better reintroduce it. Our objective was to observe the resources of the game in the context of

1 This is the interdisciplinary research program *Polisoma* "Du somatique au politique" (2015–2018), directed by Fabienne Martin-Juchat (Pr. in ICS, GRESEC, UGA), Thierry Ménissier (Pr. in Philosophy, MIAI Grenoble Alpes, UGA) and Valérie Lépine (Pr. in ICS, LERASS, UM), part of the research action "Emotions, communications and organizations: contemporary organizational mores" within the GRESEC Laboratory, Université Grenoble Alpes.
2 This is evidenced by the number of publications on the subject (Fernandez et al. 2006, 2008; Lhuillier 2006; Loriol 2012; Roux 2013; Gravereaux and Loneux 2014; Bonnet 2020).

collective support for occupational health prevention. The aim was to see to what extent a prevention method that integrates games, through the shifts it makes, is likely to encourage the expression of emotions in care staff and to recreate a work group within care units that are in difficulty or even suffering.

In this presentation, we will focus on the field experiments that we were able to conduct in a long-term care unit (*Unité de soins de longue durée*, USLD), as part of an initial exploratory investigation. The USLD is a geriatric accommodation center which takes care of elderly, polypathological residents requiring continuity of care. Firstly, we will explain the research methodology used, based on a collaborative and participatory approach. Then, we will detail the method of prevention through play which was implemented with the nursing staff of long-term care units. Finally, we will present the first results obtained in the context of this exploratory survey on the benefits of the preventive method implemented with groups of caregivers.

1.2. Methodology of the research

1.2.1. *Collaborative research and participatory methodology*

Based on the observation that there is a lack of support for healthcare workers with regard to the emotional work (Hochschild 2017) that they carry out in order to deal with various emotional situations, which are sometimes difficult in their care of patients, and also of families and carers, it seemed interesting to us to pursue a field experiment on the subject, which is based on a partnership and collaborative approach. Indeed, as the Information and Communication Sciences (ICS) researchers, Valérie Lépine and Fabienne Martin-Juchat state on the subject of collaborative research:

> through co-operation with practitioners, researchers gain access to knowledge that is empirically nourished by practice and, consequently, theoretically more complete in terms of understanding the role and characteristics of *praxis*. In other words, co-operation with actors makes it

possible to avoid banalities, naiveties, simplicities or simplifications due to a lack of knowledge of the field (Lépine and Martin-Juchat 2020).

Partnership research, in a collaborative mode between researchers and practitioners, also offers the possibility of co-producing knowledge and methods, through exchanges and sharing that are likely to lead to the emergence of a community of practice (Lépine and Martin-Juchat 2020).

With this in mind, we developed a research methodology based on a co-construction approach that combines and crosses our perspectives as researchers and practitioners. Our objective was to observe, within the hospital institution, the possibilities of supporting the emotional work of the caregivers within the framework of prevention interventions in occupational health. We developed a method of occupational health prevention that integrated the use of games to encourage the emotional expression of caregivers and to discuss their work with groups. Numerous research studies in the social sciences show the benefits of discussing work in order to give professionals the "power to act" (Clot 2010, 2021). However, we are forced to note the limits of such spaces of expression, with the "power to act" being reduced to a "power to say" (Jolivet 2014), due to organizational resistance in the introduction of real structural changes expected by employees in terms of the environment or working conditions (Dumas 2018, 2019a). In a similar vein, ICS researcher Olivia Foli shows the paradox of a widely solicited expression of employees within organizations, even though they feel little (or not at all) listened to, which tends to be explained by the misuse of such expression spaces. Indeed, they remain largely instrumentalized within the organization, inscribed in standardized and rigid managerial frameworks (Floris 1996; Olivesi 2006) giving rise to a restricted, regulated, constrained expression when it is not censored and not allowing for the possibility of "real words" (Foli 2018, p. 341). Yet, as the researcher stipulates, expression promotes creativity at work, which itself participates in the preservation of health: "creativity is an operator of health and with it, intrinsically, the communicative processes that allow it to be deployed in the individual and collective experience of work" (Foli 2018,

p. 334). It is in this capacity that the game in the prevention method we present here was mobilized.

In support of these studies and observations, we introduced a research methodology that was at the heart of the development of the prevention method implemented. Indeed, we have carried out several field observations conducted within the framework of group support in which the prevention method in question was deployed. On the basis of these observations, both participatory (on the practitioner's side who carried out the prevention interventions) and non-participatory (on the researcher's side), the prevention method using the game was thus led to evolve, by progressive enrichment, according to the results observed both from the point of view of the relational and affective dynamics as well as of the creative and reflexive resources that could emerge from the group in the forms of support introduced. We present here the exploratory survey stage that we conducted in 2020 with the nursing staff of a long-term care unit.

1.2.2. *Exploratory survey in the USLD: some elements of the organizational context*

Our field survey was held in the geriatric service of the USLD, which includes more than 80 professionals for 64 residents. We chose to conduct our exploratory research stage in this department, which was marked by strong discontent among the teams. Historically, the teams of this service moved in 2004 to a new building, which gave rise to numerous strikes as soon as it was put into service to denounce poor working conditions that did not allow for quality care (lack of equipment, lack of personnel, too large a structure, etc.). The teams experienced a high turnover, which also affected the local paramedical and medical hierarchy. In addition, the nursing staff were confronted by a lack of increase in numbers despite the change in patient profiles, with an increasingly high dependence level, a source of an increase in the burden of care and a workload more and more centered on basic care (hygiene, food, etc.), to the detriment of technical care and especially relational care. However, it should be noted that the possibilities for organizational changes remain dependent on the tripartite agreement between the university hospital, the departmental council and the regional health agency (*Agence régionale de santé*, ARS), leaving little room for maneuver and little possibility of acting in terms of staffing levels.

The service also encounters difficulties from the point of view of the attractiveness of the position, due in particular to strong depreciative representations linked to geriatrics, which remain associated with situations of abuse. Thus, there is a polarization in the profiles, with a proportion of caregivers who owe a length of service to the institution and are therefore obliged to work in said department, and others who have chosen their place of practice as well as the geriatric specialty. However, the lack of knowledge and recognition of this specialty tends to generate frustration and even anger amongst the nursing staff, which accumulates if there is no possibility of transforming it into action (service projects, organizational changes, etc.).

At the beginning of 2020, the teams were facing a very deteriorated work situation with an experience of interpersonal harassment, in a context of major absenteeism (more than 50% of caregivers), which tended to generate extreme power issues in the distribution of overtime. Indeed, the caregivers who agreed to carry out covering shifts were paid overtime, which could even double their salaries. Within this competitive environment, communication was proving deleterious in the team, which was opposed to each other, clipped and could no longer share information about patients. Because of this organizational context, occupational health prevention interventions with care professionals were proving to be complex, as team turnover made it difficult for a preventive approach to take hold. Caregivers were confronted with both the physical burden of care (numerous handling operations, manipulation of residents to provide care to polypathological patients) and the psychological burden: the profile of the dependent patient, who may present cognitive disorders, required them to think about assisting the resident due to their impending death, which was rarely discussed within the team.

Our exploratory investigation, carried out within the service, consisted of three long observation periods conducted during occupational health prevention support programs (between January and March 2020) which enabled the prevention method implemented to be deployed. These field observations gave rise to a logbook and were the subject of a condensation of the "raw" data collected (Huberman and Miles 1991) so that, on the one hand, we could progressively focus our gaze over the course of the interventions carried out in an observational approach that became attributive (Blanchet et al. 2005) and, on the other hand, to enable the development of a more precise analysis grid in view of a second phase of field investigation extended to other departments and other teams within the hospital institution. Moreover, this exploratory survey phase, which was part of a process of co-production of knowledge and methods, based on a cross-fertilization of our views, was an important step in the development of the prevention method implemented.

1.3. The use of games as a method of occupational health prevention

The use of the game[3] was designed to facilitate access to a reality that is too brutal for the teams, given the risk of seeing exchanges degenerate and become more like the settling of scores between individuals. When used as part of collective occupational health prevention support, the game provided a "framework" that makes it possible to approach the issues differently by mobilizing new resources among the staff. While such recourse is not innovative in itself, the game nevertheless constituted an innovative medium for questioning and discussing work and its organization within the hospital institution, a fortiori from the singular angle of the affective dynamics at stake.

This method of prevention through games was implemented in two stages, which we will present here. In the first stage, the collective support was carried out by the prevention worker using the Dixit® game. The cards in the game were used to encourage staff expression, as the rules of the game themselves were not followed (Mousnier et al. 2016). The cards offered different images whose evocative power

---

3 Game resources have been the subject of many works that we cannot develop here. We refer here in particular to the article by Di Filippo (2014), which recontextualizes the theories relating to play by Johan Huizinga as well as by Roger Caillois.

could lead to projecting feelings, similar to photolanguage. The caregivers were invited to choose at least one card from the deck and to tell the others the reasons for their choices based on their professional experiences. The verbalization of affective experiences was then reinvested within the collective exchanges, in order to encourage both listening and empathy: the aim here was to bring the collectives together to discuss the work, to confront their perceptions and even to apprehend the work from another angle. All 84 cards were laid out for the team to see, and each person had to then silently select one to three cards to illustrate, firstly, the current communication within the team and, secondly, the changes they would like to see in this team communication. This was followed by a random round of discussion, without any obligation on the part of the rest of the team or even the prevention worker who was facilitating the support. In the second stage, the Concept® game was used, this time following the rules of the game (apart from the counting of points): the aim was to make people guess an object, a character, a film, etc., using the images proposed on the game board[4]. In this case, the prevention worker introduced into the discussion professional situations that the team could encounter and that were sources of conflict. It called upon symbolic resources to encourage discussion of certain values, certain emotions and certain experiences, shared or not, in any case little evoked or even trivialized within the team. The objective was thus to allow the team to communicate differently by resorting to the expression of each person's representations in order to promote intercomprehension. The discordances emanating from the group mainly concerned the professional practices in the ways of taking care of the residents. The chronicity of the patients, linked to the fact that the USLD represents their last place of life, tended to generate a strong attachment between the caregivers, the residents and even the residents' families and constituted a specificity of the patient's care. The harmonization of practices within the care team thus inevitably requires team communication, which must be maintained and adapted so that the caregivers can exchange information on therapeutic activities and initiatives that each of them can set in motion around the patient.

---

4 To make a guess, caregivers could place several counters on the game board with "concepts" (represented as pictures) they could choose.

The game is a medium that tends to encourage people to speak out and to include the other in the exchange. It tends to divert the conflict and tensions inherent in the organizational constraints evoked in professional situations. This prevention method, which uses games, puts the team's questions about work back into perspective, in the light of the triptych self/other/work organization.

1.4. Results of the exploration and experimentation stage

1.4.1. *Contributions of the game: gaps and displacements*

Our field observations with the nursing staff of the long-term care unit show that the use of games in occupational health prevention support tends to displace the "framework" of the hospital institution, in the Goffmanian sense of the term. Sociologist Erving Goffman (Goffman 1991) distinguishes two main categories of experience frameworks: natural frameworks and social frameworks. While natural frameworks are related to the order of the physical world, laws of nature so to speak, social frameworks are similar to human constructions that correspond to common rules shared by individuals. Each social framework responds to a set of rules that are specific to it. The sociologist enriches his approach by distinguishing between primary and transformed frameworks. He defines the primary framework as "one that is seen as rendering what would otherwise be a meaningless aspect of the scene into something that is meaningful" (Goffman 1991, p. 30). The primary framework, whether it belongs to the natural or social one, is therefore part of the ordinary, familiar framework, which is self-evident for individuals who experience it daily without questioning it. The framework is thus a form of prior knowledge for understanding the situation which is validated in the interaction. However, for Erving Goffman, a transformation of the primary framework can occur, which is then similar to a modalization:

> I refer here to the set of conventions by which a given activity, one already meaningful in terms of some primary framework, is transformed into something patterned on this activity but seen by the participants to be something quite else. The process of transcription can be called keying.

Goffman goes on to say

> My choice of term – "key" – has drawbacks, too, the
> musical reference not being entirely apt, since the musical
> term "mode" is perhaps closer to the transformations
> I will deal with (Goffman 1991, p. 54).

So, we will continue to use the term "modalization" rather than
"keying".

The transformed framework thus resembles the primary framework
but differs in certain respects, the central element being the point of
view of the individuals taking part in the framework in question. It is
then either a "modalized framework" in the case where the
transformation of the framework is achieved explicitly for the
individuals or a "fabricated framework" when the displacement of the
framework takes place voluntarily but without the knowledge of the
participants, in particular with a view to creating disorientation within
their actions. In other words, modalization is "a transformation that is
not hidden" (Goffman 1991, p. 283), as opposed to "fabrication",
which is not said.

By supporting occupational health, there tends to be a
transformation of the primary framework of the order of modalization,
sometimes on the borderline of manufacture. The introduction of the
game itself creates a departure from the logic of the work and the
framework of the hospital institution. This modalization of the
framework through the use of the game tends to shake up the members
of the nursing staff, as reflected in the shared astonishment they
showed at the start of the prevention interventions when they were
presented with the modalities of the game. As we observed in our
exploratory survey, the game can then allow for a redistribution of
roles within the group in the space of exchange and sharing which it
creates between members. Once they were familiar with the "rules"
and the cards, the pleasure of the game tended to win over the
participants, thus influencing the affective and, consequently,
relational dynamics of the group. Indeed, among the staff members,
forms of "letting go" could be observed, of the order of affective
impulse, in relation to the affective staging of themselves observable in

the context of work inscribed in the logic of control. Such deviations were manifested in the participants, who found themselves won over by the excitement, caught up in the game of "competition". In this respect, it should be remembered that the games chosen, whether Concept® or Dixit®, are based on the sharing of representations, in a process of intercomprehension; in other words, the "winners" are those who manage to approach and even grasp the modes of representation of the other in their relationship to the work and to the team. From the point of view of the affective dynamics at stake, the displacements observed participated in forms of the suspension or even the logics of self-control in force being forgotten in the hospital institution, thus transforming the intervention framework of the order of manufacture (Goffman 1991). In support of this observation, it is interesting to note that this displacement of the framework of affective experience, in the deviations it creates, can prove destabilizing, uncomfortable and even embarrassing both for the nursing staff accustomed to more "classic" modes of intervention and for the prevention worker. Because organizational affective rationalizations are powerful (Dumas 2019a, 2019b), affective expressions considered unusual within the institution act as "infractions" (Goffman 1974), which can generate a sense of transgression and fear of loss of control, which is difficult to shake off.

On the basis of these initial observations, we wondered how the contributions and resources of the deviations and displacements to support the reflexivity of the group with regard to relational and affective dynamics in the work could be reinvested.

1.4.2. *The game to approach the relational and affective dynamics within the construction of the caregiver and the work group*

Faced with the discrepancies and shifts observed within the group, the role of the prevention worker was to mirror to the caregivers, the affective and relational dynamics created by the game, in order to show different forms of relationships with others and possible dialogues. The objective was to support the caregivers in the implementation of a reflexivity towards the affective experiences within the work team. In support of the game's resources, one of the challenges was to question and discuss the work through a roundabout way. At each stage of the game, the aim was to move forward with the group on the blocking points encountered in the work. In the suffering and/or conflict-ridden groups that we observed, the use of the game, through the images and stories it provided, allowed the participants to reveal themselves while keeping themselves and the other at a distance, and to find points of contact to discuss sensitive or even violent subjects collectively. The expression of emotions on the part of the nursing staff was thus achieved by circumvention effects, by progressive disclosures, which also made it possible to avoid, to a certain extent, the reactivation of certain conflicts between people and the exchange of ad hominem attacks within the group, participating in an ethics of discussion (Habermas 1987) favorable to the establishment of a collective, as the following extracts show[5].

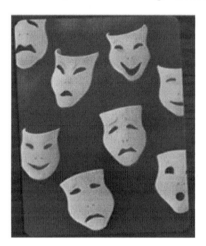

Figure 1.1. *Card from the Dixit® game*

It represents moods. The team is decisive in terms of moods, mine and others. The most important thing here is everyone's mood and it's pretty oppressive (quote from a state-registered nurse (SRN), excerpt from the logbook, first observation time, January 2020).

---

5 These excerpts were accompanied by the cards selected by the caregivers who explain their choice here.

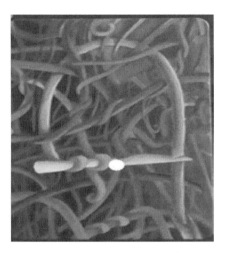

Figure 1.2. *Card from the Dixit® game*

I chose the knife with the jungle because that's the feeling I have, that there's a lot of intractable stuff and I don't know if we're going to get out of it. But the knife comes to cut the curse (a health executive, from the logbook, second observation time, February 2020).

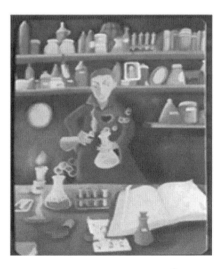

Figure 1.3. *Card from the Dixit® game*

I took the same card as last time: always the same vision. Every time we work together, sometimes the recipe is a success, sometimes not, sometimes it's harmonious and sometimes it turns into a nightmare. When we are at work, we have to create chemistry and sometimes it can explode (an SNR, extract from the logbook, third observation period, March 2020).

The role of the prevention worker also involved showing the caregivers the influence and implications of the work environment, the organization of work and the working conditions in the emotional and relational problems encountered by the team. The challenge here was to put the figure of the caregiver and that of the work group into discussion within the team with a view of showing the way in which both are constantly co-constructed. It was also a question here of shifting the commonly shared representations of conflict situations encountered within the teams, associated with people and not with work organizations. The challenge was to show the implications of work in the tension of teams in order to recreate a benevolent collective. Here again, the aim was to reposition work in the space of exchange and sharing, making it a "place of relationality" (Meunier 2007) which encourages the recreation of links. The game can therefore be used to mediate individual and collective reflection on professional practices in order to provide caregivers with new resources that are useful for recreating a work group that can initiate organizational changes within the hospital institution. For example, during the observation of the prevention method through play, tensions emerged within the team of care assistants (CAs) regarding the distribution of snacks to patients. The lack of standardization of practices made it possible to initiate the development of a reference system (regarding patients' tastes and preferences) created by the team itself and made accessible to all of the nursing staff.

The use of games can allow for the (re)establishment of spaces for exchanges on work within teams in distress, whose members tend to withdraw into themselves and are no longer able to call upon the resources of the collective. One of the challenges is then to put into words the professional experiences that are obstacles in order to make them intelligible, representable and shareable, and thus likely to be reinscribed in the dynamics of action and change. Supported by in-depth work on the organization of work and by the management team, the use of games in occupational health prevention support can therefore promote the teams' power to act by strengthening and enriching the work groups, thus ultimately improving the quality of care for residents.

1.5. Conclusion and perspectives

Within the group support observed, it appears that games, through their recreational and also creative and participative potential, allowed caregivers to see themselves in a different light. The use of games tends to create new relational and emotional dynamics, through the expression of emotions that it can generate in the participants, which can then support reflection and reflexivity regarding the experiences within the work group. The figure of the carer thus tends to be constructed or even reconfigured through the discussion and debate of the work and the affects exchanged at work. Indeed, following this exploratory research, it appears that the use of games encourages the expression of emotions, which can be conducive to the establishment of a dialogue on emotions in the workplace, both from the point of view of the caregivers' work within the care unit and of the team's work. This first stage of exploratory investigation allowed us to refine our intervention protocol, and it is now important for us to extend our field of study to other care units within the hospital institution. Moreover, based on these initial results, our research questioning has been enriched, leading us to study the extent to which these reflexivity of affects at work, through the method of prevention by play implemented, can constitute forms of reappropriation, and therefore of resistance or even emancipation with respect to the organizational affective rationalizations in force within the hospital institution. In the course of our research, we will thus question the possibilities of emancipation developed by the caregivers, and also identify their limits.

1.6. References

Blanchet, A., Ghiglione, R., Massonnat, J., Trognon, A. (2005). *La technique d'enquête en sciences sociales. Observer, interviewer, questionner.* Dunod, Paris.

Bonnet, T. (2020). *La régulation sociale du risque émotionnel au travail.* Octarès Éditions, Toulouse.

Clot, Y. (2010). *Le travail à cœur. Pour en finir avec les risques psychosociaux.* La Découverte, Paris.

Clot, Y. (ed.) (2021). *Le prix du travail bien fait. La coopération conflictuelle dans les organisations.* La Découverte, Paris.

Di Filippo, L. (2014). Contextualiser les théories du jeu de Johan Huizinga et Roger Caillois. *Questions de communication*, 25 [Online]. Available at: https://journals.openedition.org/questionsdecommunication/9044.

Dujardin, P. and Lépine, V. (2018). Quelles compétences et ressources pour les cadres de santé dans la gestion des situations à forte charge émotionnelle ? *Santé Publique*, 30(4), 507–516.

Dumas, A. (2018). Prévention de la santé au travail et politiques d'information et de communication des entreprises : le transfert de responsabilité et mutations de l'espace public. *Les Enjeux de l'Information et de la Communication*, 19/3A [Online]. Available at: https://lesenjeux.univ-grenoble-alpes.fr/2018-supplementA/06/.

Dumas, A. (2019a). La prévention de la santé et de la sécurité au travail comme dispositif de médiation de pratiques collaboratives : enjeux et limites. *Communication & Organisation*, 55 [Online]. Available at: https://journals.openedition.org/communicationorganisation/7824.

Dumas, A. (2019b). Des compétences communicationnelles à la régulation des émotions au travail : les rationalisations organisationnelles que révèle l'étude des dispositifs de prévention de la santé en entreprise. *Communication et Management*, 1, 65–77 [Online]. Available at: https://www.cairn.info/revue-communication-et-management-2019-1-page-65.htm.

Dumas, A. and Pavillet, J. (2018). Méthode visuelle et dynamiques affectives des cadres de santé autour de l'hôpital d'aujourd'hui et de demain. *Revue française des sciences de l'information et de la communication*, 14 [Online]. Available at: https://journals.openedition.org/rfsic/4029.

Fernandez, F., Lézé, S., Marche, H., Steinauer, O. (2006). Émotions, corps et santé : une politique de l'émoi ? *Face à face*, 8 [Online]. Available at: http://faceaface.revues.org/224.

Fernandez, F., Lézé, S., Marche, H. (2008). *Le langage social des émotions. Études sur les rapports au corps et à la santé*. Économica, Paris.

Floris, B. (1996). *La communication managériale – La modernisation symbolique des entreprises*. PUG, Grenoble.

Foli, O. (2018). Médier la parole sur l'activité : une dynamique de créativité au cœur des enjeux de santé au travail. *Actes du 21ème Congrès SFSIC*, 2, 331–343 [Online]. Available at: https://www.sfsic.org/wp-inside/uploads/2020/05/actes-vol-2-congres-sfsic-2018.pdf.

Goffman, E. (1973). *La mise en scène de la vie quotidienne 1. La présentation de soi*. Éditions de Minuit, Paris.

Goffman, E. (1991). *Les cadres de l'expérience*. Éditions de Minuit, Paris.

Gravereaux, C. and Loneux, C. (2014). Risque et acteurs au travail TIC et dislocations des relations. L'exemple d'un nouveau dispositif numérique (SIH) dans un centre hospitalier privé. *Communication & Organisation*, 45 [Online]. Available at: https://journals.openedition.org/communicationorganisation/4503.

Habermas, J. (1987). *Théorie de l'agir communicationnel*. Fayard, Paris.

Hochschild, A. (2017). *Le prix des sentiments. Au cœur du travail émotionnel*. La Découverte, Paris.

Huberman, M.A. and Miles, M.B. (1991). *Analyse des données qualitatives, recueil de nouvelles méthodes*. De Boeck-Wesmael, Brussels.

Jolivet, A. (2014). Promotion de la santé au travail et instauration d'un "pouvoir d'agir" : une communication de l'équilibre entre l'individuel et le collectif. *Les enjeux de l'information et de la communication* [Online]. Available at: https://lesenjeux.univ-grenoble-alpes.fr/2014/varia/06-promotion-de-sante-travail-instauration-dun-pouvoir-dagir-communication-de-lequilibre-entre-lindividuel-collectif.

Lepine, V. and Martin-Juchat, F. (2018). Situations émotionnelles de cadres de santé : les émotions au cœur de l'action et de la communication. *Revue française des sciences de l'information et de la communication*, 15 [Online]. Available at: http://journals.openedition.org/rfsic/5114.

Lepine, V. and Martin-Juchat, F. (2020). Enjeux communicationnels des recherches partenariales dans le contexte des *open labs*. *Communiquer*, 30 [Online]. Available at: http://journals.openedition.org/communiquer/ 7396.

Lhuillier, D. (2006). Compétences émotionnelles : de la proscription à la prescription des émotions au travail. *Psychologie du travail et des organisations*, 12, 91–103.

Loriol, M. (2012). *La construction du social. Souffrance, travail et catégorisation des usagers dans l'action publique*. Presses universitaires de Rennes, Rennes.

Martin-Juchat, F., Lépine, V., Aznar, M. (2018a). L'agir affectif dans le travail d'encadrement : un objet de recherche interdisciplinaire. *Revue française des sciences de l'information et de la communication*, 12 [Online]. Available at: http://journals.openedition.org/rfsic/3471.

Martin-Juchat, F., Lépine, V., Ménissier, T. (2018b). Émotions, dispositifs et organisations : quelles finalités, quels engagements, quelles dynamiques ? *Revue française des sciences de l'information et de la communication*, 14 [Online]. Available at: http://journals.openedition.org/rfsic/3795.

Meunier, D. (2007). La médiation comme "lieu de relationnalité". Essai d'opérationnalisation d'un concept. *Questions de communication*, 11 [Online]. Available at: https://journals.openedition.org/questionsdecom munication/7363.

Mousnier, E., Knaff, L., Es-Salmi, A. (2016). Les cartes Dixit comme support aux représentations métaphoriques : un média d'intervention systémique sous mandat. *Thérapie familiale*, 37, 363–386.

Olivesi, S. (2006). *La communication au travail. Une critique des nouvelles formes de pouvoir dans les entreprises*. PUG, Grenoble.

Roux, A. (2013). Rationalisation des émotions dans les établissements hospitaliers : pratiques des soignants face à un travail émotionnel empêché. *Communiquer*, 8 [Online]. Available at: http://journals. openedition.org/communiquer/227; DOI: 10.4000/communiquer.227.

2

The Digital Space as a Resource for Accessing an Alternative Discourse of Caregivers on Caregiving

This chapter is part of the ACCMADIAL project devoted to the experiences of caregivers of patients diagnosed with Alzheimer's disease. The analysis of interviews in relation to media and legal discourses allowed us to identify some of the representations of caregiving from the point of view of institutional actors. However, the apparent homogeneity of these dominant discourses was crossed by other voices, notably those of caregivers, who testify to different affiliations which are specifically analyzed in this chapter.

In order to study this hypothesis of a muted discourse, an alternative or counter-discourse, to which the digital world – thanks to its singular relational dynamics – could provide a space for expression, we have constituted a corpus of blogs whose authors are the caregivers themselves. Through an analysis situated in the field of discourse analysis that combines a quantitative textometric approach and a qualitative enunciative approach, the aim is to study how, through these linguistic practices, caregivers construct themselves, (re)define their status and roles, how they position themselves in relation to the discourse of traditional and/or legitimate actors, and what solutions they adopt to maintain, or even better, live their support.

2.1. Introduction

This contribution is part of the ACCMADIAL project devoted to the experiences of caregivers of patients diagnosed with Alzheimer's

Chapter written by Nathalie GARRIC and Frédéric PUGNIÈRE-SAAVEDRA.
For a color version of all figures in this book, see www.iste.co.uk/corroy/patients.zip.

disease. While the caregiver has been and often remains in the shadow of the Alzheimer's patient and Alzheimer's disease[1] itself, this research is entirely dedicated to the concept of caregiving. To this end, we have centered the project on a corpus of interviews that functions as a reference corpus at all stages of the analysis: in other words, with regard to corpus linguistics, all data collected in the project is correlated with this corpus, in particular to construct our descriptions and interpretations of caregiving.

Therefore, at the beginning of this project, we posed the existence of a socio-discursive reality that testifies to the existence of certain actors, the caregivers, with an experience that we wanted to know more about because it is the object of political and legal discourses, as well as of health discourses that testifies to its actuality. The experience also testifies to the complexity of this status, particularly the hypothetical vulnerability it grants to those supporting the patient, especially in the context of Alzheimer's disease, which 1) affects the elderly and 2) relates to a neurodegenerative disorder.

The analyses of the interviews in relation to the media and legal discourses enabled us to identify some of the representations of care from the perspective of the institutional actors. But the apparent homogeneity of these dominant discourses was crossed by other voices, notably those of caregivers, testifying to different affiliations which we will specifically analyze. In this chapter, because of the interventionist objective of the ACCMADIAL project, we are interested in the figure and experience of the caregiver as constructed by the main actors of caregiving, and in particular we will question the existence of an alternative discourse to the institutional discourse, or a counter-discourse (Moïse and Hugonnier 2019) to this discourse, as constructed and maintained by the media.

---

1 See our previous work, in particular Garric et al. (2020), which shows that the reference to the caregiver is quantitatively much less than that to the disease in the media space.

2.2. The caregiver: a suffering social figure whose status has recently been recognized

Two moments structure this status (see Figure 2.1): from 2001 to 2011, civil society actors were mobilized to set up plans, Alzheimer's charters and ethical reflection groups. From 2015 to 2020, the legislative period in France gradually led to the recognition of the caregiver status with the law of December 14, 2015, known as the "ASV" *law for the adaptation of society to aging*, which is based on three pillars: anticipation of loss of autonomy, overall adaptation of society to aging and support for people who are losing their autonomy. This law expresses the ambition of a global adaptation of society to aging, mobilizing all public policies: transport, urban development, housing, etc. It prioritizes support in the home.

This 2015 law also defines the family caregiver as "a non-professional person who provides assistance on a principal basis, full-time or part-time, to a dependent person in their family, for the activities of daily living". According to the website of the French Ministry of Solidarity and Health[2], this regular assistance can be permanent or non-permanent and can take several forms, including: nursing, care, support for education and social life, administrative procedures, coordination, permanent vigilance, psychological support, communication, domestic activities, etc. Two years later, leave for *caregivers* was introduced and the law recognized the *caregiver status*.

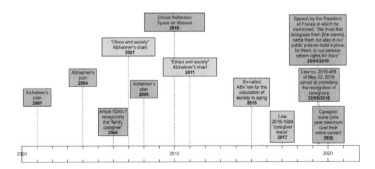

Figure 2.1. *Timeline of key events on the caregiver status*

2 See: https://solidarites-sante.gouv.fr/.

According to a 2020 Crédoc study[3], family caregivers are developed as a pillar in the caregiving relationship, but are nevertheless part of a form of suffering with a posture of fragility and sacrifice:

> They compensate alone for the fragility and loss of autonomy of their loved one or come in addition to professional help. The use of professionals is most often initiated by caregivers because of fear or refusal to perform intimate acts such as washing or changing clothes (48%) and because of a lack of time, especially for young and future retirees. Although professional help is most often used when the frailty of the person increases, it does not replace the intervention of family caregivers, who remain the mainstay of support of the cared-for person in his or her home.

> [...]

> These caregivers in fragile situations are older, alone in helping, in greater financial difficulty and in poorer health than other caregivers. Occupied by the material or moral assistance they provide, caregivers forget themselves in this relationship. The impact on their social life and health is significant. More than one in two caregivers have to make sacrifices: 62% have given up seeing relatives or going on vacation (49%). 60% have had to change their work schedule, take time off work (61%) and anticipate retirement (54%) to care for their loved one. 31% feel their health has deteriorated compared to last year, with future retirees seemingly the most affected. The oldest retirees, who are caregivers for their spouses, express more strongly a feeling of sacrifice and isolation (Crédoc/Cnav, May 2020).

---

3 Source: CRÉDOC/CNAV, quantitative survey "Aidants" – Futurs retraités et retraités du régime général, May 2020.

2.3. A digital field constructed in correlation with a reference corpus of caregivers' words

We were led to question the existence of a discourse other than the institutional discourse, such as how it is constructed and maintained by the media by an initial observation, in part already oriented by our first results, namely from the media corpus. We will try to find out whether the digital space, in particular blogs, could pose a challenge to the "hierarchy of seeing" (Voirol 2005a, pp. 18–19) if digital devices such as the forum and the blog participate in constructing a counter-discourse and if these digital texts of intimate testimonies are part of exteriority as defined by Casilli (2013) "[exteriority] as a practice of exposing or unveiling oneself intended to consolidate and appropriate one's image as well as to increase one's social capital".

Before focusing on the study of certain blogs and forums, we conducted a preliminary search on *Google* and on *Qwant* using the following four keywords: *blog, forum, aidant* [French for caregiver] and *Alzheimer*. We only retained the first 20 occurrences for each of the search engines considering that information relegated to page 2 is information not consulted and not read.

	Google	Qwant
Promotional communication for health, insurance, nursing home investment groups	1	1
Good practice guide: advice, recommendations, verbal advice, practical advice	9	9
Promotion of companies offering personal services	3	2
Blog/forum	2	1
Press article	4	5

Table 2.1. *Searches for the keywords* blog, forum, aidant, Alzheimer *on Google and Qwant. For a color version of this table, see www.iste.co.uk/corroy/patients.zip*

On the one hand, the results obtained show that, regardless of the browser used, the figure of the caregiver is used as a social figure to produce a discourse on good practices (institutional discourse) and, more marginally, to refer to singular expressions made by caregivers in blogs or forums: platforms for creating websites and blogs such as overblog.com and wix.com. On the other hand, they show that digital devices do not necessarily offer a space of visibility to develop an alternative speech since they are located in a very distant position by the search engines. We then shifted the focus to these digital corpora to study what they put into words.

We constituted the following corpus in an attempt to respond to our working hypotheses with a digital corpus comprising 9 blogs/forums[4] (caregivers' statements) relating to caregivers of patients diagnosed with Alzheimer's disease. We found that, as in the case of media discourse, caregivers' speeches are quoted most frequently. The examples are particularly numerous, and the quotation appears even when our search included the keywords "testimony" or "word" of a caregiver[5]. The "free" speech of caregivers seems to be rare: the first site we came across was the blog of Colette Roumanoff, a caregiver for her husband, who has published several books on illness and caregiving. Two sites were created: *Bien vivre avec Alzheimer* and *Alzheimer autrement*, which welcome caregivers' testimonies which we have completed with the testimonies of *Avec nos proches*.

We compare this digital corpus to a reference sub-corpus of individual interviews spaced 6 months apart (time for reflexivity) with three caregivers and to a sub-corpus of interviews with two families (spouse and/or all children) also spaced 6 months apart to describe, compare and interpret the data.

---

4 See: https://www.carenity.com/forum.
http://regini.over-blog.com/ (Vivre avec une maman Alzheimer).
https://uneplume-desmots.over-blog.com/.
https://aucoeurdeloubli.forumactif.org/.
https://www.ghislainebourque.ca/blogue.
https://www.journalduneaidante.com/.
http://www.alzheimer-autrement.org/temoignages.php.
http://www.bienvivreavecalzheimer.com/.
https://passionsetraisons.blogspot.com/search?q=Alzheimer.
5 See: https://www.femmeactuelle.fr/sante/sante-pratique/maladie-alzheimer-accompagner-un-proche-temoignage-aurelie-36934.

Type of corpus	Number of forms	%
Digital media (blog/forum)	35,479	9.1
Individual interviews	121,509	31.3
Family interviews	231,692	59.6

Table 2.2. *Distribution by type of corpus and percentage*

2.4. Theoretical framework

This research is situated in the French tradition of discourse analysis, thus, starting from discourses, we analyze caring as a practice that constructs a socio-ideological reality in the space of circulation of words. Here we posit that every social reality is a construction in the form of practices and leads to a discursive production constructed in the relationship of discourses proper to different communities (interdiscourses) that convey and produce representations and values by their way of saying. In other words, caring is defined as a discursive object:

> [...] that is, objects that are constructed, proposed, negotiated, modified, rejected or ratified in and through discursive processes. Discourse objects, as the term indicates, have a discursive mode of existence: it is in and through discourse that they emerge contextually and are transformed dynamically (Mondada 1995, p. 57).

In this socio-constructivist perspective, certain discourses belonging to certain communities are dominant because of their influence, volume, media propagation, the legitimacy of their authors, as well as their discursive and linguistic strategies, omnipresent to the point of defining a norm, a doxa, while others are dominated and heard in silence: "whole sections of social experience remain in the shadows and silence, condemning from then on situations, experiences, actors and practices to remain on the margins of public attention" (Voirol 2005b, p. 99). The latter are no less real, they also inform us about the reality of assistance, but they do so from the point of view of the weak actor, in the sense of being *weakened* by words, representations and values of the other. However, discursive objects are characterized by their instability (Mondada 1995), since their way of life is interactive, they encounter new dialogical paths that can change power relations so that the division between visibility and invisibility can be questioned. In a project such as ACCMADIAL, which is both applicative and implicative, the question of care is not only a legal one, not only a recognition by name ("natural caregiver" or "family caregiver" or even "close caregiver"), we also aim to, through a work that is explicitly focused on the practices that construct care, make the discourses of the field heard through their collection, but also by making the hypothesis that some of the digital devices can offer to these weakened words singular spaces of production which are likely to modify the "hierarchy of seeing" (Voirol 2005a, pp. 18–19) through the implementation of "visibilization strategies":

> Visibility then no longer refers only to perceptual skills actualized in everyday situations but to a horizon of conflicting meanings and categorizations where contradictory definitions of "what is worth seeing" are continuously confronted (ibid., p. 19).

The discourse produced by digital devices (forums/blogs) is constitutively technologized and thus modifies the modes of writing and reading by the marks, the traces of this digital language conversion (Paveau 2017). According to Cardon and Delaunay-Téterel (2006, p. 28), the *Blog*, a contraction of the words *Web Log*, is,

> by its individual essence, a publication tool that offers people original formats for putting their personal identity into a narrative, it is also and above all a communication tool that allows for varied and original modalities of contact.

According to Marcoccia (2001a, p. 15), the "discussion *forum* is an automatically archived electronic correspondence, a dynamic digital document, produced collectively in an interactive way". Whether it is a question of the *forum* or the *blog*, the question of mastering language technostructures and recognition by peers is essential: "One cannot be a blogger without obtaining the recognition of other bloggers" (Cardon and Delaunay-Téterel 2006, p. 68). This is an essential condition for the sustainability of these sites; they are maintained if they are read, reread and quoted, if their content is of interest to other Internet users.

The various digital devices thus offer new spaces likely to modify the order of traditional media; this idea is today defended by many researchers, especially but not exclusively with regard to militant practices. However, it should be emphasized that these devices have no de facto visibilization potential. They can also constitute a place where the representations, values and meanings of traditional media can be reproduced. However, their hegemony can also be challenged, creating difficulties due to another discourse that resignifies the object and destabilizes the dominant interpretations. To qualify this other discourse, we distinguish, with Moïse and Hugonnier (2019, p. 124), "the counter-discourse [which] is constructed in a lively and emotional argumentative opposition, between refutation, confrontation and questioning, that can reactivate the arguments or even the attacks of the source discourse" from the alternative discourse where "it is not a question of countering head-on the arguments of the first discourses, […] but of bringing, through life experiences, another vision of the world".

We will approach the corpus with a double entry: a quantitative approach using a few textometric tools (*Lexico 3, Tropes, Le Trameur* and *Iramuteq*) which allow access to indices built in contrast to the established sub-corpora and a qualitative approach for an analysis aimed at the discursive stakes of the characteristics, in particular enunciative, specific to each community.

2.5. Some results

2.5.1. *The caregiver: an actor who receives little attention in the media and political arena*

The issue of caregiving is not absent from the discourses of the public sphere; it is addressed in Macron's program, the law of 2005, revised by the Law of Adaptation of Society to Aging of 2015. It has endowed caregivers with a legal existence, consolidated by Law No. 2019-485 of May 22, 2019. Nevertheless, if we consider the emergence of the term "caregiver" in journalistic discourse, we realize that its entry is late, that it is often linked to the coverage of legal texts and that, although it was introduced in the discourses devoted to Alzheimer's disease, it remains very largely in the background. This observation has been confirmed in the discourses of recent years.

In fact, we have carried out searches of the French national press using the *Europresse* archive since 1944. We found 8,521 occurrences of the term "Alzheimer", which dropped to 680 when the term was associated with "*proche*" meaning relative or close family member (which can refer to either the caregiver or the person being cared for) and to 170 when it was associated with "*aidant*" (caregiver). The term "caregiver" is therefore only marginally representative of the context of the disease. This frequency difference is represented in Figure 2.2 which compares the curves of the three previous surveys.

It was in 1987 that mention of the disease was introduced, taking off from the year 2000 which led to the Alzheimer's plans, *Plans Alzheimer* 2001, 2004, 2008. Three years show remarkable usage: 2007, 2008 and 2011. They can be hypothetically correlated with institutional initiatives: *Charte Alzheimer éthique & société* (The Alzheimer's Ethics & Society Charter) 2007, 2011, *Espace de Réflexion Éthique sur la Maladie d'Alzheimer* (Ethical Reflection Space on Alzheimer's Disease) in 2010 (AREMA). Although the French term for "caregiver" was used from 1996, the name "caregiver(s)", then in quotation marks, first appeared in 1999. The French term for "relative(s)" appeared from 1998 to refer to the patient's close circle, without excluding the reference to the patient themselves. The gap between the curves is an indication of the essentially medical and scientific, even legal, coverage of the disease. Although the caregiver is considered in the texts dealing with the disease, they are generally proportionally only very little the object of the discourses: putting the illness into words does not establish the carer as a reference, or does so only marginally.

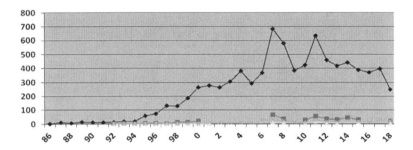

Figure 2.2. ■ *Frequency of the word "Alzheimer"* ■ *Frequency of "Alzheimer" + "Proche"* □ *Frequency of "Alzheimer" + "Aidant"* □ *Frequency of "Alzheimer" + "Accompagnement" (support) (Lexico)*

A top-down hierarchical analysis or dendrogram, which consists of a contextual lexical form of processing intended to show the main themes by word classes, of this media corpus confirms the previous observations. We identify three classes (classes 4, 3, 2) which refer to an institutional and societal processing of the disease and its management by three themes: medical-associative, labor code and dependence towards the community. A fourth class is constructed, which refers singularly to the treatment of the disease from the point of view of the family unit, which is integrated into the media discourse through the reported speech.

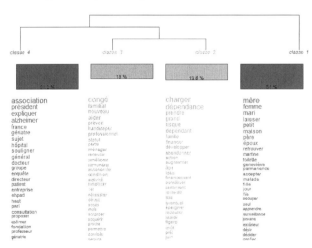

Figure 2.3. *Dendrogram of media discourse (Iramuteq)*

From this interpretive background briefly presented here, we focused on studying this muted speech that seemed to be heard in class 1.

2.5.2. *A strong singularity of the digital corpus in a positive dimension*

As a first step, we conducted an exploration of the digital corpus using correspondence factorial analysis[6] (see Figure 2.3), which led us to restrict the initially selected sites to a few that were in close proximity. This analysis shows that the sites that come together are those carried by an authority, in this case literary[7], except "*Avec nos proches*" which proposes a "wall of testimonies" integrated into the corpus and a non-integrated blog close to that of "*Aidons les nôtres*", which is also not integrated. This exploration also shows that four sites, *Carenity* (forum, advice), *La maison des aidants* (mood posts), *Le journal d'une aidante* and *vivre avec une maman Alzheimer* (blogs by anonymous individuals), are rather distant from those grouped on the right of the horizontal axis, represented by a red circle, maintaining a certain homogeneity. The latter are characterized by a very strong practice of reblogging, known as "reported technodiscourse repeating" (Paveau 2017). This practice contributes to the construction of their coherence and imposes itself as an index of community cohesion. We reduce the textometric explorations to the following corpus.

---

6 A correspondence factor analysis (CFA) is a family of statistical methods of analysis that is applied to tables of numbers and summarizes approximately all the information contained in the starting table by a few series of numbers [LEB 94].

7 Roumanoff, C. (2015). *Le bonheur plus fort que l'oubli*, Points; (2017). *Alzheimer: accompagner ceux qu'on aime (et les autres)*, Librio; (2019). *L'Homme qui tartinait une éponge*, La Martinière (eds). Bourque, G. (2017). *Et si perdre la tête rapprochait les cœurs*, Médiaspaul. Vilain, L. (2017). *L'envol d'un père*, Le livre de la plume.

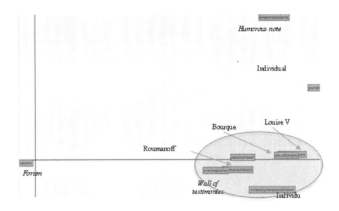

Figure 2.4. *CFA of the digital corpus (Lexico)*

The interview corpora and the digital corpus were first analyzed using top-down hierarchical analysis. We constructed the dendrogram of each sub-corpus to compare it and to access some general interpretation elements.

While the corpus of individual interviews evokes four semantic groupings with priority given to the daily life of the caregiver and the patient, then to the relationship with medicine and the disease, followed by life stories and placement in a facility (see Figure 2.5), the corpus of family interviews evokes, for its part, three semantic groupings with the expression of the daily life, then the disease and the life story (see Figure 2.6).

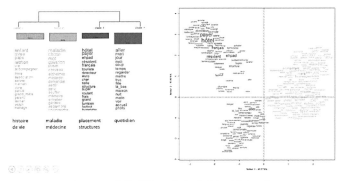

Figure 2.5. *What do individual interviews reveal through a dendrogram (Iramuteq)?*

We note that the question of placement in a facility is less likely to arise in the case of caregivers where the entire family (the caregiver spouse and children) participates, because the relay is more sustainable in its implementation.

The digital corpus reveals different semantic constructs in which the placement structures are not so much evoked as the life stories and future perspectives with the disease in a very positive way.

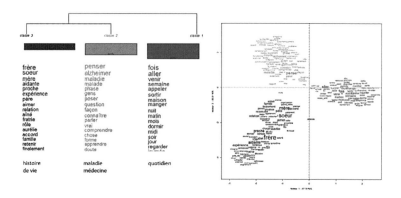

Figure 2.6. *What do family interviews reveal through a dendrogram (Iramuteq)?*

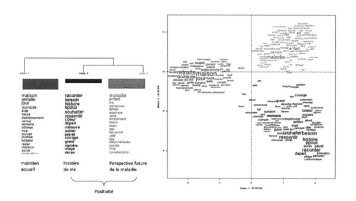

Figure 2.7. *What does the digital corpus reveal through a dendrogram (Iramuteq)?*

When comparing the two interview corpora with the numerical corpus, notable differences appear at the level of frequent word categories[8], except for the opposition connectors, which are highly represented in each of the sub-corpora and which we will discuss below.

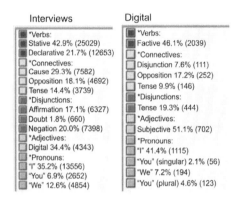

Figure 2.8. *Word categories by corpus (Tropes)*

We observe that the digital corpus is much more anchored in actional realization, temporal modalization and subjectivity: the caregiver thus narrates the support activities that they share with a loved one with positive emotions while inscribing them in daily life and frequently in iteration.

Anonymous example 1:

> As for me, I go to see her every night after work. She knows. We eat our soup together. She has a good appetite. Very often, we give her a plate or I give her mine. It is also true that at noon, she sometimes eats nothing or almost nothing. She does not stay in one place, she gets up from the table […] When she sees me arrive

---

8 The identification of frequent word categories is a feature offered by the *Tropes Zoom* software. It compares the frequency of word categories of each analyzed text with a database consisting mainly of literary texts and some media texts to formulate a judgment of conformity or over-representation.

in the evening, or in the afternoon on weekends, I am welcomed by her extraordinary smile, and very often by a love that radiates from her heart. And the hugs, the kisses. And often she tells me with passion things that are incomprehensible. But I listen to her with great interest (Source: Vivre avec une maman Alzheimer)[9].

These results are refined by the analysis of specificities. It involves studying the terms that are particularly over-representative or under-representative of the sub-corpus in terms of relative frequency. We can see that the numerical corpus evokes the disease with a largely positive specificity (sp. +65) (see Figure 2.9) in its optimistic and/or reassuring side with a positive specificity (approximately sp. +20) of the lemma *live* (see Figure 2.8). Moreover, we note a strong anchoring in the benevolent emotional universe (see Figure 2.10).

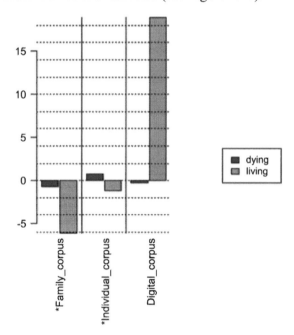

Figure 2.9. *Specificities of dying and living by corpus (Iramuteq)*

---

9 See: http://regini.over-blog.com/.

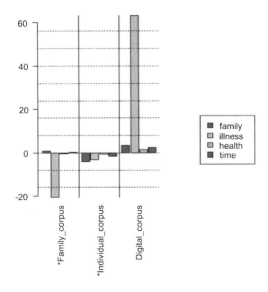

Figure 2.10. *Family, illness, health and time specificities by corpus (Iramuteq)*

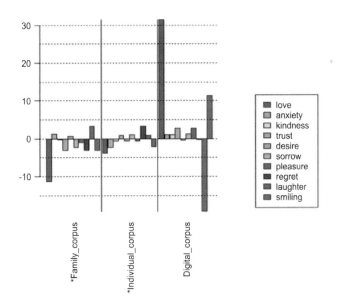

Figure 2.11. *Specificities of emotions by corpus (Iramuteq)*

2.6. Division and/or continuity of the caregiver status constructed by blogs

We continue the analysis by focusing on certain markers with an enunciative function that will enable us to more precisely study the positioning of the discourses studied in the arena of discourses, their relationship(s) with others and in particular to the doxa and their status in the public space.

If we look at the specificities of the interlocutionary relationship, we note a dominant use of the personal subject pronoun "I" (*je*), which is co-constructed with the pronoun "one" (*on*) in the corpus of interviews, whereas it is co-constructed with the pronoun "we" (*nous*), which refers to the family, the caregiver/care receiver couple and, by extension only, the caregivers (community) or, more rarely, generic statements in the digital corpus.

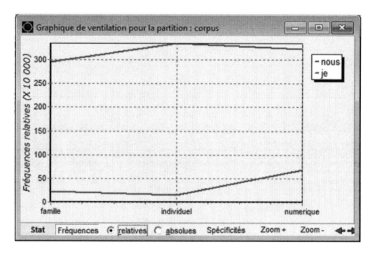

Figure 2.12. *Breakdown of "I" (je) and "we" (nous) pronouns in French by corpus (Lexico)*

While "the interpretation of the pronoun *one* is often underspecified, as it is the referential expression preferentially associated with a group of people with blurred boundaries" (Landragin and Tanguy 2014, p. 124), "we" is interpreted much more precisely, here with an exclusive value that constructs a speaker as in communion with the cared-for (example 2) or with their family (example 3), in this case a party, which defines the caregiver of this alternative discourse that Moïse and Hugonnier (2019, p. 125) define as "having to express a concrete truth and objectified emotions, to touch his or her audience"[10]. The commitment of caregivers as a profoundly humanistic act in intimate and singular care leads to its presentation in its ideal dimension.

Anonymous example 2:

> We dance, like before, even if now he doesn't move his legs much, we make funny faces and we laugh. [...] I know that time is short. In the last few years, we have been rushing to make the trips, weekends with our loved ones, etc. that we promised ourselves to do more of when we retired. In addition to all our happy years, Michel is now teaching me the serenity of living in the moment. We savor together all that we can still "take" from life.

Anonymous example 3:

> I don't understand the "we don't have a mother anymore but an Alzheimer's patient" reflections. My husband and I have been living with Mom for the past 6 months, and Mom has learned new things. She has adapted to our way of life, and is 81 years old.

We also note a very high specificity (sp. +6) of "carer(s)" in the digital corpus, whereas the term is very low (specificity close to 0) in the interview corpora (see Figures 2.12 and 2.13). The same is true for the specificity (sp. +52) of the expression of possession followed by the French reflexive pronoun "me", which reinforces the construction

---

10 In the article in question, the authors mention a fourth condition that involves distancing themselves from homophobic hate speech, since their contribution deals with it: *Discours homophobe. Le témoignage comme discours alternatif.* We consider that in our case, this last condition is not operative.

of a tightly knit community ethos as presented by Cardon and Delaunay-Téterel (2006, p. 17):

> The interface of the blog must then be seen as a repertoire of contacts allowing individuals to connect with others around statements through which they continuously and interactively produce their social identity.

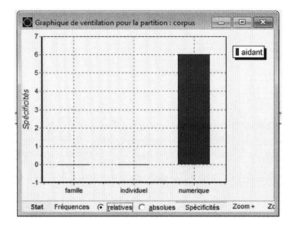

Figure 2.13. *Breakdown of the French word for "caregiver" (aidant) by corpus (Lexico)*

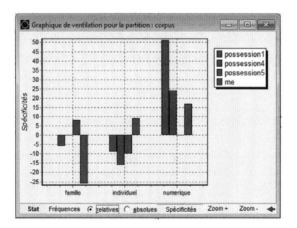

Figure 2.14. *Breakdown of possession markers and the French personal complement pronoun "me" (Lexico)*

Finally, we conclude the comparative analysis of our corpora by turning our attention to the oppositional connectors in *Tropes*. The frequency readings show that the two corpora studied use the oppositional relation in comparable propositions. However, a closer look at the distribution of these markers reveals a fundamental difference: "even if" and "yet" are singularly over-represented in the numerical corpus, while "but" is strongly underemployed.

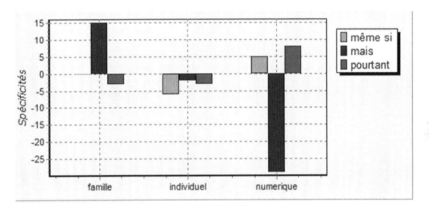

Figure 2.15. *Breakdown of oppositional–concessive connectors: even if (même si), but (mais), yet (pourtant) (Lexico)*

"Even if" (*même si*) and "yet" (*pourtant*) are operators of the concession. The latter designates an enunciative operation that establishes a relationship between two propositions. One supports an argument, the other a counter-argument that restricts or destroys the validity of the first. According to Morel (1996), the concession is divided into three types in discourse: "1) logical concession, 2) restrictive concession, 3) argumentative concession." Let us look at some excerpts:

Anonymous example 4:

> Every day that passes is a day saved from being put in a nursing home. I love taking care of her. **Even if it is true** that she is constantly demanding and that, in the long run, I break down.

Anonymous example 5:

> [...] after I stopped working last March, **even if** the beginning was difficult, after a few months, we found a pace of life, she and I.

In examples 4 and 5 (to be completed with example 2 above), "the concessive subordinate is presented as having been previously asserted by another enunciator" identifiable in the dominant voice with which the speaker is thus in agreement. The two propositions can thus exist simultaneously thanks to the conjunctive group: the speaker expresses the positivity of the helping activity while relativizing it by an argument shared with the general opinion.

Anonymous example 6:

> It is a strange disease, one that makes you forget names but not faces, your current address but not that of your first house, that makes you butter your sandwich with a knife and not with a spoon, that makes you open the door of the dressing room instead of the toilet, that makes your words incoherent **yet** that allows a mother to say to her son: you are a good boy, come and give me a kiss.

Anonymous example 7:

> On the other hand, the dementia, the delusions, the hallucinations, the obsessive behavior, I can't handle it. It's unbearable. **And yet**, when she is peaceful or asleep, I forget that I have so many times almost called the ambulance to take her to the psychiatric hospital's emergency room.

In examples 6 and 7, "yet" also marks a logical concessive relationship which, while acknowledging the counter-argument constituted by knowledge about the disease and the difficulty of helping the patient, makes it possible to justify the persistence of the support. While the speaker expresses his agreement with the suffering of the carer, he simultaneously expresses his disagreement with public health policies by refusing the placement.

2.7. Conclusion

The construction of a digital corpus of caregivers' words enables us to access a singular discourse on support. This discourse exploits some of the properties of the digital device and blogs in particular: it seems that the notion of extimacy makes it possible to construct the self as a form of statement, but this one struggles to express itself without the community support that finds its strength in a figure of affiliation benefiting from a certain legitimacy thanks to the literary practice. The claim based here on writing justifies further research on the role of narrative as a resource for living, perhaps better living, the caregiving role.

The discourse constructed in this way escapes certain normative constraints on the experience of caregiving as presented by the media and legal discourse. It integrates certain indices that express a positioning in the interdiscourse of the different communities approaching care without, however, introducing a strong opposition between them, even more so by sometimes seeking a space of conciliation between the points of view.

Thus, this discourse is constructed within and for a very restricted, almost private community, which makes it an alternative discourse that does not reach the role of a counter-discourse. The very low representation of the blogs studied, their relatively weak reach in the public space because it is limited to family, private or even intimate experience, does not allow this alternative discourse to free itself from the circulating discourse (doxa). The hierarchy of the blogosphere is maintained, and the discourse does not extend beyond the community, perhaps indicating that caregiving is seen by its actors as an activity that is by definition internal to the family, a family affair that finds positive feelings, and which does not wish to be externalized under the evaluative and standardized gaze if it is to receive public recognition.

2.8. References

Cardon, D. and Delaunay-Téterel, H. (2006). La production de soi comme technique relationnelle. Un essai de typologie des blogs par leurs publics. *Réseaux*, 4(138), 15–71 [Online]. Available at: https://www.cairn.info/revue-reseaux1-2006-4-page-15.htm.

Casilli, A. (2013). Contre l'hypothèse de la "fin de la vie privée". *Revue française des sciences de l'information et de la communication* [Online]. Available at: http://journals.openedition.org/rfsic/630 [Accessed 16 November 2021].

Garric, N., Pugnière-Saavedra, F., Rochaix, V. (2021). Construction langagière de la figure de l'aidant du malade d'Alzheimer : dénominations et mise en mots interdiscursive dans les pratiques. *Corela*, 18–1, 2020, 25 June 2020 [Online]. Available at: http://journals.openedition.org/corela/11302 [Accessed 12 July 2021].

Landragin, F. and Tanguy, N. (2014). Référence et coréférence du pronom indéfini on. *Langages*, 3(195), 99–115. doi:10.3917/lang.195.0099.

Lebart, L. and Salem, A. (1994). *Statistique textuelle*. Dunod, Paris.

Marcoccia, M. (2006). L'analyse conversationnelle des forums de discussion : questionnements méthodologiques. *Les Carnets du Cediscor*, 8 [Online]. Available at: http://journals.openedition.org/cediscor/220 [Accessed 8 June 2021].

Moïse, C. and Hugonnier, C. (2019). Discours homophobe. Le témoignage comme discours alternatif. *Semen*, 121–136, hal-02014526.

Mondada, L. (1995). La construction discursive des objets de savoir dans l'écriture de la science. *Réseaux*, 13(1), 55–77.

Morel, M.-A. (1996). *La concession en français*. Ophrys, Paris.

Paveau, M.-A. (2017). *L'analyse du discours numérique. Dictionnaire des formes et des pratiques*. Hermann, Paris.

Tisseron, S. (2011). Les nouveaux réseaux sociaux : visibilité et invisibilité sur le net. In *Les tyrannies de la visibilité. Être visible pour exister ?*, Nicole, A. (ed.). Érès, Toulouse.

Voirol, O. (2005a). Présentation. Visibilité et invisibilité : une introduction. *Réseaux*, 129–130(1–2), 9–36 [Online]. Available at: https://www.cairn. info/revue-reseaux1-2005-1-page-9.htm.

Voirol, O. (2005b). Luttes pour la visibilité. Esquisse d'une problématique. *Réseaux*, 129–130(1–2), 89–121 [Online]. Available at: https://www. cairn.info/revue-reseaux1-2005-1-page-89.htm.

3

Co-design with Patients with Chronic Diseases for Information and Training Materials Related to Connected Implants

In order to improve heart failure management, the European Institute of Innovation and Technology (EIT Health) is financing for three years a multidisciplinary and multi-stakeholder research project on a connected implantable device named "MyHeartSentinel". Thanks to this subcutaneous implant, the objective is to detect heart failure aggravation from the patients' cardiorespiratory data, and therefore adapt their treatment as soon as possible to avoid emergency hospitalizations.

For the human and social sciences team, the key challenge is to involve patients in the development of digital supports about the implant. In particular, it is about co-designing a study with a small team of patients as collaborators, in order to integrate the future monitored patients' needs in education and training. We brought together these patients to assist us not only in designing the study aiming at identifying the patients' needs, and also in following the development of the digital application which will provide services linked with the connected implants. During our interviews, we used affect stories that focused on their healthcare experience, in order to bring out collective and organizational dynamics involved in heart failure management.

3.1. Introduction

Heart failure is a serious and disabling chronic disease that progresses gradually, especially if left untreated. It occurs when the

Chapter written by Ambre DAVAT and Fabienne MARTIN-JUCHAT.

heart is no longer able to circulate enough blood in the body: as a result, the patient gets out of breath quickly and feels very tired during exercise, which greatly limits activities. Although young people can develop heart failure, for example, following a heart attack, the vast majority of patients are elderly, often suffering from several other comorbidities such as hypertension or diabetes. As a result, heart failure is the leading cause of hospitalization in people over 65 years, and some studies estimate that as many as one in five people will develop heart failure in their lifetime (The Heart Failure Policy Network 2018).

One of the main challenges in monitoring heart failure is the prevention of cardiac decompensation: a sudden worsening of symptoms, which requires emergency hospitalization and can lead to sudden death. One approach currently being considered to prevent these cardiac decompensations is to set up remote monitoring devices, which record the patient's physiological parameters and alert the medical team if there are any signs of deterioration in the patient's health. There are both non-invasive devices, such as connected scales, and implantable devices: for example, a pacemaker records cardiac data, which can either be downloaded during an annual consultation with a rhythmologist (a cardiologist specializing in heart rhythm disorders, electrical activity of the heart and cardiac prostheses) or be monitored remotely on a more regular basis. Several clinical trials have already taken place to test these different devices (Desnos and Jourdain 2020). However, the results of these studies are contradictory: some conclude that remote monitoring does, indeed, reduce mortality, hospitalizations or patient symptoms, while others measure no significant effect between the remote monitoring group and the control group. This may be explained by the fact that there are significant variations not only in the technology used, but also especially in the way telemonitoring is implemented, particularly with regard to the degree of patient involvement and their specificities being taken into account.

Our research, in cooperation with the "Ethics & AI" Chair of the Grenoble MIAI's 3IA Institute[1], is taking place in the framework of RealWorld4Clinic, a European consortium funded by EIT Health[2] which aims to develop a new connected monitoring implant to improve heart failure monitoring and which brings together researchers from different disciplines and private and public actors. One of the ambitions of the humanities and social sciences team is to address the ethical, legal and social issues related to the emergence of implant-monitored health, by adopting a patient-centered approach. In particular, one of the components of the project[3] is to co-design with heart failure patients the information and training devices intended to present the project to future patients by integrating their training and information needs. In particular, a digital mobile application will be developed that will allow patients to have feedback on their remote monitoring and access to their health data.

The objective of this chapter is to detail the original method that we have developed, which consists of co-designing the study (problem, hypotheses, methodology) with a group of patients, based on their narratives of the affects that have marked their course of care. This chapter presents both the theoretical and methodological framework that justifies the interest of co-designing with patients based on affect stories, and its application in the RealWorld4Clinic project. In conclusion, we will come back to the ethical and societal stakes of co-designing technological innovations with patients in the health field.

3.2. Co-design based on affect stories

Co-design is the development of technological objects or services in collaboration with their future users. It encompasses a large number

---

1 Institut pluridisciplinaire en intelligence artificielle MIAI@Grenoble Alpes: ANR-19-P3IA-0003.

2 European Institute of Innovation and Technology.

3 As this project has many aspects (social, medical, legal, financial), the questions relating to the protection of personal data in connection with the implant are dealt with in their own right in another part of the study and will therefore not be the focus of our discussion.

of collaborative practices, which have developed simultaneously within different design disciplines (Zamenopoulos and Alexiou 2018). In the healthcare field, this co-design can take many forms depending on the levels and types of involvement of the different stakeholders (especially patients and care staff) (Slattery et al. 2020). The methods used are also very diverse: one example is the toolkit proposed by the Auckland District Health Board (Boyd and McKernon 2010).

Several co-design studies have already been carried out in the case of heart failure, notably to develop or improve a mobile application intended to help patients monitor their treatment (Triantafyllidis et al. 2015; Grosjean et al. 2019; Woods et al. 2019) or to design a procedure to address the end-of-life issue with patients and their families (Hjelmfors et al. 2018). Most often, this involves designing the desired object iteratively with a small group of patients, care staff and providers, following a method suggested by the researchers.

The originality of the method we propose is that it consists first of co-designing the study aiming at developing information and communication devices with a small group of patients, based on their stories of affects in relation to their care pathway. This method of collecting patients' experiences allows us, in a few sessions, to construct a very detailed representation of the main issues in relation to the actors involved (carers, relatives, associations, industrialists, researchers), the technology (relationship with the body, with the data collected, with monitoring, with follow-up) and the disease (between acceptance and adaptation), and to put forward hypotheses in relation to the research.

First, three to six "patient collaborators" must be recruited: these people have to be able to speak in a group, and be willing to support us throughout a university health research. The objective is to define with them the main areas of questioning of the study, and then to validate the hypotheses as well as the methodology used to test them with a larger and more representative sample of patients. They are also asked to discuss the results of the interviews and to validate the analyses proposed by the researchers.

Concerning affect stories, we ask the people interviewed to tell us about their care experience, emphasizing the major positive or negative emotions, the way in which their relations with their care staff and their entourage have changed as a result of the disease, and how an implant could be part of a dynamic of acceptance and/or adaptation to the disease. The objective is to let the participants express themselves as freely as possible, avoiding orienting their testimony by our conceptions a priori, in order to familiarize ourselves with their vocabulary and to let the major areas of questioning and difficulties encountered appear. When used in a group interview, the affect stories also create a sense of being together, which facilitates the expression of major issues related to a problematic situation, methodological choices and the formulation of solutions (Martin-Juchat et al. 2018; Martin-Juchat 2020; Nicogossian et al. 2021).

3.3. Application to the RealWorld4Clinic project

3.3.1. *Constitution of the group*

To create the group of patient collaborators, we first contacted Résic38: the network of heart failure patients in Isère. This is not a network of patients, but a network of health professionals, located at the Grenoble University Hospital. It is run by a multi-professional team, responsible for organizing the care pathway of patients referred to them on discharge from hospital. Their approach, based on therapeutic patient education, is based on negotiation, the aim of which is to adapt medical orders to the lives and expectations of patients. Résic38 regularly organizes training sessions on heart failure for health professionals, as well as group education sessions for patients who are members of the network.

Thanks to Résic38, we were able to recruit three patients with good communication skills, ready to share their experiences on their care pathway and to follow the development of the project:

– Olivier*[4], 56 years old, former director of medical-social establishments;

– Michel*, 73 years old, former occupational physician;

---

4 First names have been changed.

– Henri*, 76 years old, former executive in the construction industry.

Olivier* and Michel* are particularly involved in the network and are recognized as "resource patients": they are trained in therapeutic education, regularly take part in group education sessions and participate in writing the network's newsletter. Henri* has no particular status within the network. However, he is very involved in the group therapeutic education sessions, which he continued to attend remotely during the pandemic.

Subsequently, a fourth person agreed to join the co-design group:

– Sylvie*, 50 years old, lawyer.

Sylvie* lives outside the Grenoble area and was contacted because of her activity on social networks. Unlike the other participants, she has never received therapeutic education through a formal network, but communicates regularly with other patients.

3.3.2. *Course of the sessions*

Each group session lasted approximately two hours. They took place by videoconference once every three weeks, and were recorded with the agreement of the participants. The exchanges were not transcribed in full, but we noted certain verbatim extracts, when they related directly to the experience of heart failure or to the relationship with the carers. These verbatim quotes were sent individually to each participant by e-mail. In addition, a summary was written at the end of each session and sent to the participants, along with any documents presented during the session. In the following, we will present the course of the first four working sessions that led to the development of the study methodology.

3.3.3. *Identification of issues through affect stories*

The main part of the first session consisted of an affect story: the participants had to recount, one after the other, their care pathway, from the first signs of the disease to the present day. They were instructed to emphasize the major emotions they felt, as well as their relationships with care staff and with their family, friends and professional environment. Finally, we proposed a personification exercise of the disease: they had to describe their relationship with heart failure by imagining that it was embodied by a person or an animal.

Through these affect stories, we were able to identify broad areas of questioning related to implant-based remote monitoring. These are presented in Figure 3.1, along with the hypotheses developed thereafter.

3.3.4. *Main questions and development of hypotheses*

The analysis of the first session as well as our bibliographic research allowed us to develop several hypotheses, which we presented to our patient collaborators during a second group interview. Their comments allowed us to validate and refine these hypotheses, particularly with regard to heart failure monitoring.

Indeed, based on the affect stories, we had initially assumed that the primary interlocutor of heart failure patients was their cardiologist. However, during this second session, the patient collaborators insisted on the fundamental role of the general practitioner (GP), whom they see much more regularly, and perceive as the "coordinator of their overall health". They saw the GP as having a holistic view of the patient, as opposed to the single-organ view of cardiologists: in particular, the GP must be able to adapt the specialists' recommendations on a case-by-case basis so that they can be lived with by their patients. In addition, the patient collaborators suggested that neither cardiologists nor general practitioners have the time to provide therapeutic education to their patients, with the assumption that they lack training: this is therefore done by nurses, for example, in the framework of the Asalée program. Thus, instead of a patient–cardiologist duo, we have identified an ideal care team, whose main actors are the cardiologist, the attending physician and the therapeutic education nurse.

3.3.5. *Development of the method*

In a third meeting, we proposed several methodological avenues to the patients in order to test these hypotheses:

– additional interviews with heart failure patients to better understand the diversity of the pathways;

– interviews with patients who already have cardiac implants to identify the anxieties experienced and the points of vigilance requiring more information;

– interviews with health professionals to better understand the impact of the system on the care pathway and the place of therapeutic patient education in practices and training.

We also discussed how to recruit study participants (patients and healthcare professionals).

Subsequently, and in view of the difficulties of recruitment, we chose to give priority to interviews with patients. Only a few informal interviews were conducted with health professionals.

3.3.6. *Review of the study's progress*

Once the research method was validated with the patients, we began to implement it. Session 4 consisted of feedback on the initial progress, and asking for their analysis of some of the observations from the literature and the new interviews. We also introduced the theme of the following sessions: the collaborative development of information and communication materials related to the implementation and its follow-up. In particular, it is planned to co-design therapeutic education sessions related to the implant, as well as a mobile application allowing patients to access their follow-up data.

LEGEND:
in bold underlined: additions/corrections made by patient collaborators
✓   Hypothesis confirmed after additional interviews
❖   Hypothesis to be confirmed

Are there any patient profiles for which the implant
is (or is not) appropriate?

In particular, is it necessary for the patient to have "accepted" their disease in order to
be able to enter into a telemonitoring approach?

✓   Rather than profiles, it is a matter of modeling a temporality in the acceptance of
the disease.

    ✓   It is according to this temporality that the presentation of the implant
by the care team and the services associated with the implant must be
thought out.

        ❖   The implant can be an additional means of reassuring the
patient and helping them to enter into a process of
acceptance/adaptation to the disease.

    ✓   **The existence of a patient network would be a considerable help in
addressing patients' fears, supporting them in their adaptation to
the disease and training them in the use of digital tools.**

What are the decisive factors that would cause a person to accept/reject a monitoring
implant?

✓   The decisive factor is the relationship of trust with **the care team.**

    ❖   This depends on the training of care staff in therapeutic patient
education.

        ❖   Therapeutic education of the patient conditions acceptance of
the disease.

What are the main sources of anxiety
related to cardiac monitoring implant
placement?

✓   **Risks related to the operation**
      (pain, infection)

❖   Risks related to personal data
      (cybercrime, insurance refusal)

✓   The consequences on daily life
      (visibility of the implant, body sensations, constraints)

✓   The consequences on the relationship with the medical team
      (loss of social ties)

> **What would be the impact of a monitoring implant
> on the care pathway?**

✓   Remote monitoring of heart failure via implants requires the appearance of new actors.

    ✓   They may be healthcare actors responsible for overseeing health data, **or technical consultants responsible for solving IT problems.**

✓   The implant must be associated with monitoring services for patients (e.g. mobile application). These monitoring services must allow patients to:

    ✓   have access to their health data

    ✓   better understand their disease through an objectification of symptoms

    ✓   embody the privileged link of patients with their care team

Figure 3.1. *Major areas of study questions and hypotheses
validated with the group of patient collaborators*

3.4. Assessment of the first phase of the study

3.4.1. *Sample*

After designing the study with our "collaborating" patients, we conducted 26 remote interviews with new patients in order to test our hypotheses.

The participants ranged in age from 21 to 89 years (average: 65 years). There were 16 men and 10 women, recruited via two health networks (Résic38 in Grenoble and the Polyclinique du Bois in Lille) or directly contacted because of their involvement in patient associations or their messages published on social networks.

Among the participants, 18 already had a cardiac implant (pacemaker or defibrillator) and 3 had worn one before receiving a heart transplant. These implants are associated with a telecardiology system, capable of automatically transmitting information concerning the electrical activity of the heart, the integrity of the implant or the battery's level of charge. In addition, 12 patients were participating, or had participated, in a remote monitoring program via connected objects: every day, they took their weight, measured their blood pressure and answered a questionnaire, the results of which were monitored by nurses. In the event of an alert (e.g. data not transmitted or significant weight gain) and approximately every two weeks if their condition was stable, these patients were called by a nurse.

Each interview lasted approximately one hour and was recorded. It began with a free-form affect story, which was then supplemented by a series of questions to explore the themes of the study. The parts of the interviews referring to affects were transcribed in full and anonymized. In the following, we analyze these interviews with respect to the hypotheses initially formulated with the patient collaborators.

3.4.2. *Patient profile/temporality in the adaptation to the disease*

We have identified a few variables that strongly influence patients' experiences.

The first is, of course, the severity of the disease. The more severe the heart failure, the more the patient is limited in their activities, because they get out of breath and tired quickly with effort. A patient with mild heart failure, who can climb stairs and carry a shopping basket, is therefore not in the same situation as a patient with severe heart failure, who has difficulty walking a few meters and carrying any load. This lack of physical ability makes the patient dependent on those around them, which can be particularly humiliating, for example, when the patient is unable to get up on their own in the event of a fall.

Moreover, two patients with the same symptoms will not perceive them in the same way depending on their lifestyle. For example, a very athletic patient will feel more limited by heart failure than a sedentary patient. The respect of sanitary and dietary rules (in particular, concerning salt consumption) is also more or less difficult, depending on the habits of each patient.

Another very important variable is age. Younger patients have difficulties in reconciling heart failure with a professional activity: they may need to be accommodated to continue their activity or to retrain, which is not always possible. If they wanted to have children, this project may be called into question because of their risk of mortality. The question of the visibility of the disease is also more acute for these patients, who suffer from an invisible disability that is often misunderstood by those around them, and which they may wish to conceal so as not to be perceived as different from others. For older patients, heart failure symptoms are often attributed to old age, which makes them more socially acceptable, and also has the disadvantage of delaying diagnosis. In addition, these patients often suffer from numerous comorbidities, which complicate their management and increase the risk of drug side effects (iatrogenesis). In some cases, heart failure can be perceived as a secondary problem compared to other diseases affecting them or their spouse: for example cancer, neurodegenerative disease, loss of sight or hearing, etc.

Finally, each course of care is different, especially with regard to the circumstances of the diagnosis. Some patients already knew they had heart disease for years before developing the symptoms of heart failure (sometimes since childhood): they were already followed by a cardiologist, and used to being limited in their physical activities. Others, on the contrary, were discovered to have heart failure from one day to the next, generally following a hospitalization. This hospitalization may have been immediate (in case of clear signs of infarction, for example) or it may have followed a few hours (or even days) of seeking second opinions. This entry into chronic illness could influence the relationship with care staff and the willingness to invest in a therapeutic patient education approach.

It should be noted that these variables are dynamic: while medical treatment can reduce symptoms and temporarily stabilize the disease, the patients' health status also tends to worsen progressively, particularly in the event of cardiac decompensation.

3.4.3. *Acceptance/rejection of implants*

Within the affect stories, cardiac implant placement is often mentioned very quickly and in a factual manner: it is through the additional questions that we were able to collect elements concerning the patients' feelings. We found that most of the people interviewed (19/21) had quickly consented to the insertion of a cardiac implant, following the instructions of their cardiologist. This is consistent with a finding by Oudshoorn (2015) regarding defibrillators: to some extent, patients have no choice because implantation is considered a standard of care and fears about implantation are outweighed by fear of death. In hindsight, the question of accepting/refusing implantation therefore does not seem very relevant, in case patients trust their cardiologist to make the best decisions regarding their health and survival[5].

We therefore looked at the reasons for trust in care staff, analyzing experiences rated positively and negatively by patients. We identified three main themes: expertise, empathy and communication skills. We thus find several fundamental competencies for therapeutic patient education. Indeed, contrary to what its name seems to indicate, this is not limited to the transmission of knowledge, but rather involves a particular approach to the doctor–patient relationship in which the doctor's role is to support the patient and help them live better with their chronic disease (Grimaldi et al. 2017). Thus, the patients interviewed appreciated care staff who managed to give them clear explanations, without medical jargon. On the contrary, the lack of

---

5 A figure much criticized by our patient collaborators and frequently put forward to underline the seriousness of heart failure indicates that the chances of survival at five years are only 50% (or even less if the article is a few years old). These easily accessible and dramatic statistics for patients do not, however, take into account age, stage of the disease or treatment.

transparency and the failure to take into account the patient's specificities was a source of tension, which pushed some people to form their own information network, among peers, to counterbalance the doctors' point of view.

3.4.4. *Sources of anxiety related to implantation*

We mainly noted existential anxieties related to heart disease, rather than to the implant itself. Thus, the patients interviewed worried about their uncertain future and regretted the loss of their physical abilities, which had a strong impact on their image and their daily life. Affects related to the implants were rarer; nevertheless, some patients mentioned the fact that the implant was a "foreign body" that would accompany them for the rest of their lives.

As expected when writing the hypotheses, we have indeed noted remarks concerning the operation, the risks, the visibility or the physical sensations linked to the implant. The question of the human link also seems essential: patients who have agreed to be monitored remotely do not see it as a substitute for face-to-face monitoring, but as a complement, an additional guarantee that they will be taken care of quickly in case of problems. It therefore seems necessary to reassure patients that telecardiology will not lead to a loss of human contact.

3.4.5. *Impact of telemonitoring on the care pathway*

We found very contrasting experiences with remote monitoring. Some of the patients were very satisfied with remote monitoring and say they felt reassured by this device: these were the patients who were being monitored via connected objects and who were contacted regularly by the program nurses, as well as some defibrillator users who had already been called in an emergency because of a malfunction of their device. Other patients, on the contrary, doubted the effectiveness of telecardiology, because they had never been called, even in case of sudden death or non-transmission of their data. Thus, as we hypothesized, it seems essential to provide dedicated telecardiology staff to establish a lasting link with patients. This is in line with the recommendations of (Pols and Moser 2009; Skov et al. 2015; Andersen et al. 2017), who have already noted the limitations of the "no news is good news" approach.

In addition, many patients found it very difficult to relate their physical sensations to their heart activity. Thus, they did not know if their symptoms were really due to their heart or to something else. At present, they have to wait for an appointment with a rhythmologist to try to make the connection between their experiences of discomfort and the data collected by their implant. Access to health data in an accessible form is therefore indeed an important issue for patients, to enable them to better understand their disease and to be involved in monitoring its evolution.

3.5. Conclusion: co-design, one of the conditions for an ethics of innovation in health?

We presented a co-design method based on affect stories and how it was applied in a European research project to develop a cardiac decompensation prevention implant. After co-designing the study method with a small group of three patients, 26 additional interviews confirmed many of the hypotheses initially formulated.

Implementing a co-design approach in a health innovation project makes it possible to respond to a pragmatic need: the aim is to develop a device that is accepted and acceptable in the daily lives of patients, based on their expectations and their experience of the disease. Moreover, we maintain that approaches of this type can be the guarantors of an ethical approach, concerned with promoting patients' rights and thinking about the societal transformations generated by new digital technologies (Béranger 2012; Ménissier 2021). Indeed, if these new connected health devices can contribute to health democracy by helping patients to better understand their disease and to better live with it, the development of predictive medicine tools could very well turn against them, by making them solely and exclusively responsible for their health (CNIL 2014).

The fundamental question is then to know if such a co-design approach with patients can have a real impact within the framework of a European research project, carried by a multiplicity of actors, and crossed by political, technical, financial and administrative stakes which exceed the capacities of recommendations of researchers in human and social sciences.

By way of perspective, we can emphasize that the main challenge of our current research (scheduled to end in December 2022) is to model the relevance and feasibility of integrating patients' experiences into the various stages and dimensions of health innovation. In the continuity of the research current called Ethical Technology Assessment (Palm and Hansson 2006; Kiran et al. 2015), it will be a question of addressing recommendations as to the way in which it is advisable to integrate the patients in the various stages and scale of development then of deployment of a health monitored by connected implants.

3.6. Acknowledgments

This publication is part of RealWorld4Clinic, a research project that has received funding from EIT Health. EIT Health is part of the European Institute of Innovation and Technology, a body of the European Union.

We would like to thank all the people involved in the project, especially those who contributed to the working group dedicated to patient information and education: Philippe Cinquin, Annabelle Drault, Raphaël Koster, Thierry Ménissier, Daniel Pagonis and Charles-Clemens Rüling.

Thanks also to the health professionals who accepted to relay our request for participants to their patients: Baptiste Barjhoux and Murielle Salvat from Résic38, as well as Jessica Dayez and Frédéric Mouquet from the Polyclinique du Bois.

Finally, a big thank you to all the participants of the study, especially the four patient collaborators.

3.7. References

Andersen, T.O., Andersen, P.R., Kornum, A.C., Larsen, T.M. (2017). Understanding patient experience: A deployment study in cardiac remote monitoring. *Proceedings of the 11th EAI International Conference on Pervasive Computing Technologies for Healthcare*, 221–230.

Béranger, J. (2012). Modélisation éthique de la recherche collaborative d'information. *Les Cahiers du numérique*, 8(1), 39–62.

Boyd, H. and McKernon, S. (2010). Health service co-design: Working with patients to improve healthcare services. *Waitemata District Health Board* [Online]. Available at: https://www.wdhb.org.nz/assets/Uploads/Documents/45f463d911/rttc_health-service-co-design-by-h-boyd.pdf.

CNIL (2014). Le corps, nouvel objet connecté. Du Quantified Self à la m-santé : les nouveaux territoires de la mise en données du monde [Online]. Available at: https://www.cnil.fr/sites/default/files/typo/document/CNIL_CAHIERS_IP2_WEB.pdf.

Desnos, M. and Jourdain, P. (2020). Télémédecine : une solution d'avenir pour l'insuffisance cardiaque ? *Bulletin de l'Académie Nationale de Médecine*, 204(8), 817–825.

Grimaldi, A., Caillé, Y., Pierru, F., Tabuteau, D. (2017). *Les maladies chroniques : vers la troisième médecine*. Odile Jacob, Neuilly-sur-Seine.

Grosjean, S., Bonneville, L., Redpath, C. (2019). The design process of an mHealth technology: The communicative constitution of patient engagement through a participatory design workshop. *ESSACHESS – Journal for Communication Studies*, 12(1), 5–26.

Hjelmfors, L., Strömberg, A., Friedrichsen, M., Sandgren, A., Mårtensson, J., Jaarsma, T. (2018). Using co-design to develop an intervention to improve communication about the heart failure trajectory and end-of-life care. *BMC Palliative Care*, 17(1), 85.

Kiran, A.H., Oudshoorn, N., Verbeek, P.P. (2015). Beyond checklists: Toward an ethical-constructive technology assessment. *Journal of Responsible Innovation*, 2(1), 5–19.

Martin-Juchat, F. (2020). Des méthodes participatives pour comprendre les dépendances au numérique et les conséquences sur la productivité. In *Pharmaphone : la voix des adolescents*, Galli, D. and Renucci, F. (eds). Deboeck, Brussels.

Martin-Juchat, F., Lépine, V., Aznar, M. (2018). L'agir affectif dans le travail d'encadrement : un objet de recherche interdisciplinaire. *Revue française des sciences de l'information et de la communication*, 12.

Ménissier, T. (2021). *Innovations. Une enquête philosophique*. Éditions Hermann, Paris.

Nicogossian, J., Heas, S., Noel, M., Misery, L., Martin-Juchat, F. (2021). Les questions que le patient atteint de dermatite atopique modérée à sévère aimerait qu'on lui pose : données d'une étude anthropologique qualitative. *Annales de dermatologie et de vénéréologie – FMC*, 8(1), A359.

Oudshoorn, N. (2015). Sustaining cyborgs: Sensing and tuning agencies of pacemakers and implantable cardioverter defibrillators. *Social Studies of Science*, 45(1), 56–76.

Palm, E. and Hansson, S.O. (2006). The case for ethical technology assessment (eTA). *Technological Forecasting and Social Change*, 73(5), 543–558.

Pols, J. and Moser, I. (2009). Cold technologies versus warm care? On affective and social relations with and through care technologies. *Alter*, 3(2), 159–178.

Skov, M.B., Johansen, P.G., Skov, C.S., Lauberg, A. (2015). No news is good news: Remote monitoring of implantable cardioverter-defibrillator patients. *Proceedings of the 33rd Annual ACM Conference on Human Factors in Computing Systems*, 827–836.

Slattery, P., Saeri, A.K., Bragge, P. (2020). Research co-design in health: A rapid overview of reviews. *Health Research Policy and Systems*, 18(1), 1–13.

The Heart Failure Policy Network (2018). The handbook of multidisciplinary and integrated heart failure care. Report, The Heart Failure Policy Network.

Triantafyllidis, A., Velardo, C., Chantler, T., Shah, S.A., Paton, C., Khorshidi, R., Tarassenko, L., Rahimi, K. (2015). A personalised mobile-based home monitoring system for heart failure: The SUPPORT-HF Study. *International Journal of Medical Informatics*, 84(10), 743–753.

Woods, L., Duff, J., Roehrer, E., Walker, K., Cummings, E. (2019). Design of a consumer mobile health app for heart failure: Findings from the nurse-led co-design of Care4myHeart. *JMIR Nursing*, 2(1), e14633 [Online]. Available at: https://nursing.jmir.org/2019/1/e14633.

Zamenopoulos, T. and Alexiou, K. (2018). Co-design as collaborative research. *Connected Communities Foundation Series*. Bristol University/ AHRC Connected Communities Programme, Bristol.

4

Institutional Communication in Healthcare Organizations as a Marker of Patient Orientation: The Case of Institutional Websites

The website: an institutional communication tool for patients

Hospitals and healthcare organizations are facing more obvious competition and a change in patient expectations that have led them to rethink their activities and find new levers for development by enhancing their offer. In this context, patient orientation as a transposition of customer orientation is expressed in the way health organizations communicate. The analysis of the websites of 17 hospitals (university hospitals, clinics and cancer centers) shows great disparities between institutions. The cultural and behavioral approaches of customer orientation appear in this particular context through the sharing of information and the setting up of specific resources and skills. In particular, the cancer center presents the most marked patient orientation through a highly developed patient information process and a personalization of the well-committed patient–caregiver relationship.

4.1. Introduction

In a world where a form of competition between hospitals and healthcare organizations is becoming increasingly evident, the ability

Chapter written by Corinne ROCHETTE and Emna CHERIF.

of these institutions to develop patient orientation (PO) is contributing to the transformation of the role given to patients and also to those who support them. This is reflected in changes in practices and in the relationship between the caregiver and the patient. PO is a lever for action that helps maintain a level of activity, as well as develop it through the enhancement of care offers and the proposal of innovative services, such as in the field of supportive care. One of the transformational challenges facing healthcare institutions is clearly their ability to assert this patient-centric orientation as a form of transposition of customer orientation (CO), particularly through their institutional communication. The objective is to further improve the satisfaction of patients as beneficiaries of healthcare services by supporting them in adopting behaviors that enable them to recover or maintain their quality of life. This objective requires paying special attention to their wishes and adopting a more holistic approach to patient care, which has long been focused exclusively on a medical approach and a passive patient posture. The key to this transformation is, among other things, the establishment of a true communication process that will allow patients (as well as their caregivers) to better understand their disease and the proposed treatments in order to express their wishes in terms of care, and that will allow healthcare professionals to develop PO that is not exclusively medical but centered on the person and their well-being. This evolution is part of a change in the care model that began a few years ago, from a biomedical approach centered on the disease to a biopsychosocial approach centered on understanding the person (Person-Centered Care – PCC) by integrating the interrelationships between the biological, psychological and social aspects of the disease (Engel 1977; Labarrière 2021). PCC is defined by the Institute of Medicine (2002) as the ability to "provide care that is respectful and responsive to individual preferences, needs, and values, and to ensure that the patient's values guide all clinical decisions". The three main objectives of patient-centered care provision should at minimum include and measure the three tenets of patient-centered care: communication, partnership, and health promotion (Constand et al. 2014, p. 8). While the patient-centered approach is expressed in the inter-individual relationship between the physician or caregiver and the patient, it can also be manifested in a more institutional way in the communication that hospitals develop towards their users.

Health organizations and specifically public institutions take advantage of their presence on the Internet to transmit their expertise to patients as they do not have the opportunity to communicate like commercial companies. Analysis of the information made available to patients on websites is a first step in understanding the PO undertaken by the institution through the way in which the relationship is envisaged: are the markers of PO identifiable? How is this expressed?

4.2. Patient orientation, between culture and behavior

The issue of patient orientation has appeared as a translation of the concept of customer orientation to the hospital sector. It is generally used as a synonym for the way in which the patient is guided through the world of medical services. In this context, the term "PO" is used as a transposition of the principles of CO to the patient and the health sector. In a context marked by competition that is not always assumed, PO is the first marker of market orientation, well before the manifestation of another of its dimensions, which is competitor orientation. Recent work shows that exhibiting a true PO helps hospitals enhance patient satisfaction (Apelian et al. 2014; Verleye et al. 2021). Patient-centeredness is manifested in the quality of interpersonal and environmental relationships. It was in the 1990s that Day (1994) defined CO as the ability to understand and meet the needs of clients. This can provide an interesting analytical basis for better understanding the manifestations of the person-centered approach and its interest. The review of the literature on CO highlights debates about the cultural or behavioral dimension (Kohli and Jaworski 1990; Narver and Slater 1990; Narver et al. 2004) that are regularly found in the healthcare sector. For example, some staff such as nurses are more patient-oriented than doctors (Verleye et al. 2020), which seems to be largely explained by the frequency of contact, which provides multiple opportunities to be attentive and to communicate, as well as by the very nature of the activity of these caregivers. Finally, beyond the organizational culture, the professional culture is not neutral regarding the presence of PO, which can be an intrinsic characteristic of certain professions, instilling their practices.

The behavioral approach (Kohli and Jaworski 1990) studies CO using observable behaviors, more precisely from "three organizational behaviors: (a) the organization-wide generation of intelligence pertaining to the nature of stakeholder communities, norms, and issues (…); (b) the dissemination of this intelligence throughout the organization; and (c) the organization-wide responsiveness to this intelligence" (Maignan and Ferrell 2004, p. 10). For Kohli and Jaworski (1990), information is central; it constitutes the heart of their conceptualization of CO. Their approach is more operational than conceptual: gathering information, sharing it and reacting to it through concrete actions. Thus, the developments in the health sector around shared and transparent information between the patient, physicians and caregivers are part of this perspective (Fossa et al. 2018).

Narver and Slater (1990) argue for the cultural approach. They argue that if CO were simply a set of activities completely divorced from an organization's underlying belief system, then it would be easy to implement market orientation (whose main component is the customer) at any time regardless of an organization's culture. However, this is not what is observed because the different dimensions of market orientation can be more or less assertive depending on the situation (p. 33). For them, culture gives rise to a set of behaviors. The organizational culture of the healthcare sector is highly singular and generally accepted as being quite different from that of the market world. As research has shown for more than 30 years, the diffusion of practices and values from the corporate world to the commercial world is a source of tension and conflict, particularly in the hospital sector (Mériade and Rochette 2022). Although the practices disseminated by the supervisory authorities over the last 30 years have been designed to transform practices by encouraging new behaviors, it can be seen that values and principles have changed little and that there is still a strong professional medical and care culture centered on technical expertise, in which practices remain deeply rooted. However, the work highlights the singularity of professional cultures. The care profession is naturally part of the care culture (care, attention, concern for the other person approached as a feeling), which differs from the cure culture, which refers more to the technical dimension, to an action that can be found in the expression of caring (Morvillers 2015).

It is therefore clear that it is difficult to separate behavioral and cultural approaches and to identify what is exclusively cultural (Bartley et al. 2007) and what is behavioral. Based on this observation, Homburg and Pflesser (2000) propose a widely validated integrative framework. This is based on the definition of organizational culture proposed by Deshpandé and Webster (1989a, 1989b), who state that an "organizational culture as the pattern of shared values and beliefs that help individuals understand organizational functioning and thus provide them norms for behavior in the organization". Thus, according to them, culture and behavior are inseparable.

PO is related in this sense to the CO, which is widely described and analyzed in the market context. In the public sector, Schneider (2016) studies the way in which the administration develops PO and its effects on internal modes of operation. In particular, he shows the interest in looking at the user's journey in order to identify the different interactions with the organization and to provide them with the means to "decode" the multiple possibilities offered by the public service through the way the organization communicates with its users (Beauquier 2003).

CO has a particular resonance in the world of healthcare. Indeed, there is a natural patient-oriented medical culture ("caring" and "curing"). However, it remains to be explored how these organizations use information to strengthen ties with patients and establish relational proximity with them. The importance of the cultural and behavioral dimensions is highly correlated with the nature and history of the organization. Private organizations naturally present these dimensions due to a strong competitive context, which seem less identifiable in a non-market world. Public organizations have been less inclined to develop CO behaviors, but to fulfill a public service mission where collective interests predominate over those of the individual. This difference leads us to wonder about the disparities in terms of the PO practices of hospitals versus clinics and about the specificity of cancer centers (Appendix, section 4.6). In fact, clinics, which are private healthcare organizations in France, are logically more familiar with the concepts of profitability and productivity than hospitals. They are generally owned by investment funds highly concerned with their profitability (such as the *Foncière Santé d'Icaden*, Gimv or Lifento Care Paneuropean). It would therefore be appropriate to postulate that their strategies are more "commercial", based on highlighting their assets and taking care of more "lucrative" patients with less complexity than those cared for by hospitals.

The objective of this study is to improve the understanding of PO by analyzing the importance given to the patient in the framework of institutional communication through the website of health institutions. The aim is to identify the behavioral and/or cultural approach of PO through the sharing of medical information with the patient (information about the stages of the patient's journey, treatments, success rates, meeting days), with the medical team (multidisciplinary consultation meetings) and the implementation of specific tools in terms of resources and skills (development of new services to meet latent needs, state-of-the-art equipment, presentation of medical teams, comfort services) or the specificities of each organization in terms of values, culture and positioning (hospitals, clinics, cancer centers).

4.3. Methodology and research proposals

To evaluate the manifestations of PO in its cultural and behavioral dimensions, we were interested in the digital communication of health organizations, more precisely in institutional websites. Two main research propositions guided our study. The first is the possibility of detecting markers of PO through the institutional communication of health institutions. The second is that there may be a difference according to the type of institution linked to their status: for-profit versus not-for-profit, institutions entirely dedicated to the fight against cancer versus institutions for which cancer care is one activity among many others (see Appendix, section 4.6). We selected an initial sample of 20 healthcare facilities based on the 2019 ranking of French hospitals and clinics published in *Le Point* magazine. Data collection was conducted during the months of May and June 2020. For this data collection, we focused on breast cancer, which is the most common cancer pathology in France with an incidence of more than 58,000 cases per year (source Institut National du CAncer, 2021). Our data collection was carried out in two stages. The first was devoted to coding data from the hospitals' digital sites (home page and the first level of the site's structure) using a summary analysis grid. Once the authors had completed the coding, an initial pooling of the data enabled the difficulties of collection and coding to be identified. A first difficulty concerned the absence of a page dedicated to breast cancer on certain hospital websites, even though they were listed in the magazine. In addition, it was necessary to distinguish between general information and information specifically focused on breast cancer. The grid was therefore refined according to the nature of the information presented (all cancers vs. breast cancer). Once this second pooling was completed, we selected 17 hospitals for which the coding process presented a uniformity of themes to be analyzed at the level of the coding grid.

Of these 17 institutions, there were three university hospitals, four private clinics and 10 cancer centers. The annual number of operations, the rate of outpatient operations and the annual number of reconstructive operations for each hospital were recorded. We performed a content analysis of each institution's website, selecting five themes:

– general data: ranking, volume of activity, reputation, nature;

– patient orientation: patient tab, patient booklet, explanation and simplification of the patient pathway, information on treatments, highlighting of specific medical services (diagnosis in one day, double consultation) and non-medical services;

– humanization of the relationship: patient testimonies, video of doctors, CVs and photos of the medical team;

– development of skills and resources: sharing of information, internal coordination, nurse coordinator, case manager, promotion of new treatments, equipment;

– evolution and adaptation of the care offer: opening of new unit(s).

4.4. Main results

The analysis of the results shows that only 6 out of 17 establishments offered a "care pathway" tab and only 3 out of 17 presented a "patient" tab on their website. We also found that the clinics were not necessarily the most vigilant on these points. Only one of the four clinics analyzed offered a "care path" tab.

General breast cancer information

We were first interested in the general and primary information offered on the institutional sites to better understand how these organizations address their patients. We found that 10 out of 17 institutions (58.82%), including one clinic and two university hospitals, made an effort to explain the pathway and stages of care, the value of diagnosis, possible treatments, etc. We also note that four cancer centers had made some efforts to simplify the pathway to make the information more accessible through its layout.

The time between the different types of care (screening, first appointment, diagnosis, intervention) was sometimes presented or highlighted (17.64%). Finally, 6 out of 17 establishments (including one clinic and one university hospital) offered information sheets and videos on care.

Detailed information on care

The efforts made by some organizations are a good initiative given the interest that this information can have for the patient in such an alarming situation. We note that only 2 out of 17 health institutions offered a presentation on breast cancer, nine attempted to explain screening and only two offered group information workshops. The clinics, with the exception of one, were not really involved in an information process for the patient. Cancer centers were also the most involved (52.94%) in providing detailed explanations of the examinations and treatments required following breast cancer screening, although further efforts are still needed. Finally, seven cancer centers and one clinic relied on the use of multidisciplinary consultation meetings to convey their expertise and only three communicated on the personalized treatment for each patient.

Information on reconstructive surgery was sometimes presented on the home page and sometimes in the "treatment or surgery" tab. A certain number of institutions invested in highlighting services such as support care (41.17%) or the explanation of follow-up after treatment (41.17%).

Highlighting specific and innovative medical services

A small number of institutions highlighted their ability to offer patient-specific and innovative medical services. Two cancer centers and two university hospitals offered patients a one-day diagnosis. Very few institutions emphasized their innovativeness, notably by highlighting the fact that they had innovative equipment (17.64%) or new treatments (23.52%). Although many institutions benefit from a historical reputation, very few use it as an advantage of expertise (17.64%). Only four cancer centers communicated on the quality of patient care.

Quality indices

In a perpetual quest for quality, public organizations, like companies, are adopting a quality approach. Health and cancer institutions are trying to measure customer satisfaction (17.64%) as well as to provide patients with certain quality guarantees through labels (23.52%), charters (5.88%), SCOPE indicators (17.64%)[1] as well as through the commitment and the place given to patients in governance committees (23.52%).

Presentation of the care team

Beyond the presence of a simple directory (52.94%), some institutions clearly understood the importance of presenting their

---

1 https://www.scopesante.fr/#/.

team. In 53% of cases, the team of doctors was presented, followed by the director of the institution (29.41%). Four institutions presented their team according to their treatment specialty and only one university hospital showed the paramedical team such as nurses, medical technicians and secretaries. It should be noted that six institutions presented photos and CVs of their care team. Finally, four institutions displayed their academic and multidisciplinary medical teams and communicated that they did not charge extra fees. Contrary to what we might have thought, it was three cancer centers and one clinic that put forward this information and not the university hospitals, probably to help demystify the representations.

Patient testimonials

Three cancer centers and one university hospital offered "patient testimonials" on the site in written or audiovisual form (23.52%). In addition, six cancer centers had a presence on social networks.

Additional information given to patients

Only three cancer centers and one university hospital offered a patient booklet. Only the cancer centers provided their patients with additional information such as accommodation possibilities (35.29%), personalized prevention units (17.64%), useful links to associations such as the *Ligue Contre le Cancer*, the INCA and Unicancer (52.34%). The presence of an "FAQ" section was noted five times, as was the presence of the booklet "*cancer mes droits*" [cancer my rights]. This can probably be explained by the strategy of the Unicancer group and the desire to highlight the uniqueness of the cancer center model, which is totally dedicated to cancer care and prevention while fulfilling a research mission.

Non-medical information

Four cancer centers and one university hospital offered their patients meeting days with other patients as well as scientific days. Only six cancer centers (35.29%) committed to offering cultural and sports activities, nutritional and aesthetic advice or personalized post-treatment support programs (supportive care).

4.5. Discussion and conclusion

Although there are strong indications of PO for all the health organizations analyzed, some significant differences persist. These differences are not in favor of the clinics, contrary to what we had postulated. It was the cancer centers and not the clinics that presented the most marked PO through a particularly developed patient information process: explanation of examinations, treatments, highlighting of expertise, innovations, etc. This indicates a strong desire to communicate with patients and encourage them to participate in the process. Furthermore, this shows a strong desire to communicate by making this information easily accessible and understandable. This is a staged presentation and clearly reflects the cultural dimension of the PO of these organizations. Thus, the use of patient testimonies, the human nature of care with a personalization of the caregiver–patient relationship, the presentation of the teams, the existence of evenings for the general public and meeting days attest to the attention paid to the relational dimension. These points are the markers of a culture of openness to the patient well-being and reveal communication practices, particularly in terms of public relations, and ultimately institutional communication practices very similar to those encountered in the commercial world. They are the means of creating both cognitive (informing, explaining) and relational (paying attention) proximity with users. We also note that university hospitals show signs of a culture that is relatively grounded in public service and the collective interest. The public service mission is an important characteristic with sites characterized by a significant informative dimension.

Our results support the observation that healthcare organizations want to strengthen patient satisfaction (Apelian et al. 2014; Verleye et al. 2020) by developing PO (Kohli and Jaworski 1990; Narver and Slater 1990), but with a more pronounced manifestation for cancer clinics. One explanation can be found in the structuring role of the Unicancer federation, which has a communications project manager and a genuine collective communications strategy designed to affirm the singularity of cancer center care by providing patients, their families and all those wishing to obtain information with easily accessible and comprehensible information about cancer. In addition, Unicancer is developing tools for the centers in the federation that contribute to the dissemination of new communication practices, for example carrying out events such as the health communication festival in which more and more institutions are participating. It is clear that communication is a means of demonstrating an evolution in organizational culture and the behaviors that result from it based on a PCC approach (Engel 1977). However, it remains to be more strongly affirmed.

Indeed, our exploratory study has some limitations, related in particular to the nature of the sample, which is mainly composed of cancer centers (10 versus 4 clinics and three university hospitals). This is related to the fact that we used a cancer pathology as the key to reading the information available on the digital sites. The specificity of the cancer centers explains their strong presence at the top of the rankings for these types of care. This study provides a closer look at the way in which PO is expressed in the organizational culture of these healthcare institutions. The behavioral dimensions are apparent in the management processes, but not very accessible with the methodology used in this study. A more precise analysis based on direct data collection from the healthcare organizations and the people in charge of their communication (management, communication department, etc.) would provide a more detailed understanding of the representation of institutional communication by the healthcare organizations, the place given to it and possibly the intentional strategy behind it.

Chapter contributions: CR developed the conceptual, theoretical framework and research question, EC and CR developed the methodology, EC extracted the results, EC and CR discussed the results. Both authors contributed to the writing.

4.6. Appendix: Terminology reminders

University hospitals are public health establishments linked to a university. They provide theoretical and practical training for future medical professionals, paramedical staff and researchers in the health sciences.

Cancer centers (CLCCs in French) are private, not-for-profit, university hospital-based health establishments that fulfill a public hospital service mission exclusively dedicated to cancer care, research and teaching. They are characterized by a model of comprehensive and multidisciplinary care for people with cancer. The *Centres de lutte contre le cancer* are united within the Unicancer group in France.

Private not-for-profit health establishments are health establishments participating in the public hospital service (PSPH). Since the law of July 21, 2009, called the "Hospital, Patients, Health, Territories" law (*Hôpital, Patients, Santé, Territoires*, HPST), they have automatically become private health establishments of collective interest (*établissements de santé privés d'intérêt collectif*, ESPIC), and as such they carry out one or more public service missions. These establishments are managed by a legal entity under private law – an association, a foundation, a congregation or a mutual insurance company. Their accounting is under private law and the profits generated are fully reinvested in innovation and the development of new services for the benefit of patients.

Clinics are private healthcare facilities. There are 1,050 for-profit establishments (clinics) with 98,522 beds (Drees)[2]. They are most often constituted in the form of partnerships or capital companies, within which the practitioners' liberal activity is exercised. From a financial point of view, the establishment contracts with doctors, whether associated or not, in order to be able to operate. Recent developments show an increasing role for external investors in private hospitalization, particularly in the form of chains of clinics that buy up existing establishments and allow for the contribution of larger amounts of capital.

2 Direction de la recherche, des études, de l'évaluation et des statistiques – the public statistical service of the French Ministry of Solidarity and Health.

4.7. References

Apelian, N., Vergnes, J.N., Bedos, C. (2014). Humanizing clinical dentistry through a person-centred model. *The International Journal of Whole Person Care*, 1(2), 30–50.

Bartley, B., Gomibuchi, S., Mann, R. (2007). Best practices in achieving a customer-focused culture. *Benchmarking: An International Journal*, 14, 482–496.

Beauquier, S. (2003). Enjeux, contraintes et potentialités des organisations "orientées clients". Le cas de deux entreprises de service : ASSUR et la RATP. PhD Thesis, Ecole des Ponts ParisTech.

Constand, M.K., MacDermid, J.C., Dal Bello-Haas, V., Law, M. (2014). Scoping review of patient-centered care approaches in healthcare. *BMC Health Services Research*, 14(1), 1–9.

Day, G.S. (1994). The capabilities of market-driven organizations. *Journal of Marketing*, 58(4), 37–52.

Deshpandé, R. and Webster Jr., F.E. (1989a). Organizational culture and marketing: Defining the research agenda. *Journal of Marketing*, 53(1), 3–15.

Deshpandé, R. and Webster Jr., F.E. (1989b). Culture d'organisation et marketing : une liste des priorités pour la recherche. *Recherche et Applications en Marketing (French Edition)*, 4(4), 25–49.

Engel, G.L. (1977). The need for a new medical model: A challenge for biomedicine. *Science*, 196(4286), 129–136.

Fossa, A.J., Bell, S.K., Desroches, C. (2018). OpenNotes and shared decision making: A growing practice in clinical transparency and how it can support patient-centered care. *Journal of the American Medical Informatics Association*, 25(9), 1153–1159.

Homburg, C. and Pflesser, C. (2000). A multiple-layer model of market-oriented organizational culture: Measurement issues and performance outcomes. *Journal of Marketing Research*, 37(4), 449–462.

Kohli, A.K. and Jaworski, B.J. (1990). Market orientation: The construct, research propositions, and managerial implications. *Journal of Marketing*, 54(2), 1–18.

Labarrière, L. (2021). Communication du chirurgien-dentiste : enquête transversale au sujet de l'orientation centrée sur la personne et du rapport au pouvoir. PhD Thesis, Université Toulouse III – Paul Sabatier.

Maignan, I. and Ferrell, O.C. (2004). Corporate social responsibility and marketing: An integrative framework. *Journal of the Academy of Marketing Science*, 32(1), 3–19.

Mériade, L. and Rochette, C. (2022). Governance tensions in the healthcare sector: A contrasting case study in France. *BMC Health Services Research*, 22(1), 1–13.

Morvillers, J.M. (2015). Le care, le caring, le cure et le soignant. *Recherche en soins infirmiers*, 3(122), 77–81.

Narver, J.C. and Slater, S.F. (1990). The effect of a market orientation on business profitability. *Journal of Marketing*, 54(4), 20–35.

Narver, J.C., Slater, S.F., MacLachlan, D.L. (2004). Responsive and proactive market orientation and new-product success. *Journal of Product Innovation Management*, 21(5), 334–347.

Schneider, O. (2016). Vers une administration orientée usager. *Pyramides. Revue du Centre d'études et de recherches en administration publique*, (26–27), 255–284.

Verleye, K., De Keyser, A., Vandepitte, S., Trybou, J. (2021). Boosting perceived customer orientation as a driver of patient satisfaction. *The Journal for Healthcare Quality (JHQ)*, 43(4), 225–231.

5

Digital Communication and Merchandising for Caregivers: The Case of Thermal Baths

This research focuses on the commercial offer proposed to family caregivers by French thermal institutions and on its stake for thermalism. To carry out this comparative study, the research combines two methods. The first compares the dedicated pages of websites of seven thermal baths and a thalassotherapy establishment offering a cure for non-professional caregivers. The second examines the views of seven actors in the thermal bathing sector through in-depth interviews. This work presents the business strategies of the thermal establishments in a niche market and questions both the approach and the place of the non-professional caregiver within them.

5.1. Introduction

Caregivers have emerged as an interdisciplinary field of research (Bloch 2012) and research work questions a societal problem that continues to grow (Caradec 2009). "The very success of the term 'caregiver(s)', which is now authoritative, testifies to this process of increasing generality to the point of now being a public cause" (Chanial and Gaglio 2013, p. 123; Charlier 2018). More specifically, Management Sciences regularly apprehend the non-professional

Chapter written by Christelle CHAUZAL-LARGUIER and Alexis MEYER.
For a color version of all figures in this book, see www.iste.co.uk/corroy/patients.zip.

caregiver, also called the family caregiver[1], through an organizational approach questioning the reconciliation of their professional and personal life (Le Bihan-Youinou and Martin 2006; Martin 2010; Domingo and Verite 2011; Piazzon 2018), and, more generally, the company (Pailhé and Solaz 2009; Belorgey et al. 2016; Gagnon et al. 2018; Charlap et al. 2019), intervening in a sensitive area that is not always one of high priority.

To our knowledge, the commercial dimension, which integrates the caregiver into a marketing approach, has not been addressed very much. However, in the field, steps have been taken. For several years now, mutual insurance companies and private insurers have been implementing actions in the provident and dependency market (Chanial and Gaglio 2013; Nabeth 2019). In this case, the commercial target may be the caregiver, seen as a prescriber (who may be a decision-maker) to adhere to a commercial offer affecting the assisted person (such as, for example, the use of personal services delivered at home) or a consumer (such as, for example, when subscribing to a service offer for the preparation of an application for financial aid to which the caregiver may be entitled). More recently, services to help caregivers (training, listening, respite, etc.) have been developed and sectors such as tourism and the spa industry, for example, have taken steps to create a commercial proposal for this target, or more broadly, the caregiver–patient couple.

The marketing approach developed by the sector of the thermalism around the close caregiver is unknown although specific because it is formulated by an actor in connection with health. Thermal establishments are

---

1 According to Article L. 113-1-3 of the French law on the adaptation of society to aging published on December 29, 2015 – "Is considered a close caregiver of an elderly person their spouse, the partner with whom they have entered into a civil solidarity pact or their cohabitant, a parent or an ally, defined as family caregivers, or a person residing with them or maintaining with him or her close and stable ties, who helps them, on a regular and frequent basis, on a non-professional basis, to perform all or part of the acts or activities of daily living".

the establishments that use on the spot or by direct adduction, for the internal or external treatment of the patients, the water of one or several regularly authorized mineral springs or its derivatives: mud or gas (article R. 1322-52 of the French Public Health Code).

Today, in addition to the conventional cures prescribed by the attending physician and reimbursed by Social Security for a duration of 18 days, the thermal establishments offer numerous short-term thermal cures known as wellness cures (also called free cures), which are not financially covered but with potential support from the mutual insurance organization and/or an allowance provided for by the law[2] and of a shorter duration (one to six days). The short-term thermal care proposed to caregivers falls into this last category. The caregiver is the target of the offer.

This communication proposes to bring responsive elements to the following question: How does the thermal establishment try to seduce the family caregiver through a specific commercial offer?

The comparative study conducted is qualitative in nature (Miles and Huberman 2003), exploratory in nature and combines a twofold methodological approach. The first is a comparative study of the dedicated pages of the websites of seven establishments and one thalassotherapy center in France, offering short-term thermal care to caregivers as shown in Table 5.1. This constitutes a restricted but exhaustive corpus in relation to the targeted offer. Indeed, only seven thermal establishments out of 109 (i.e. 6.4%) offer this short-term thermal care. The websites of the thermal establishments are the main communication supports for this short-term thermal care, which can also be relayed on specialized websites, magazine websites and, more incidentally, on some health or well-being blogs.

In order to determine the place given to this type of stay in the communication carried out on the websites, this analysis focuses on the content published on the dedicated pages (headings, types of

---

2 This type of allowance is recognized by the law of adaptation of society to aging (2015-1776) of December 2015 recognizing the right to respite.

information: Rouquette 2009). Our analysis of these Internet pages was therefore conducted around four themes: the information given on the websites, the type of discourse, the quality of the layout and the referencing of the corresponding URL. The details of each of them are proposed in Table 5.2.

	URLs of the sites
Thermal establishments	
Bagnères-de-Bigorre	https://www.thermes-bagneres.fr/quietude-programme-cible-sur-le-surmenage
Cambo-les-bains	https://www.chainethermale.fr/cambo-les-bains?gclid=Cj0KCQjwjPaCBhDkARIsAISZN7T21a3qsjwryyo3ZFaKex3nPWjC0oxnVJV1c5eGVV5rOOmQ zjK0QsaApVBEALw_wcB
La Léchère-les-Bains	https://www.balineae.fr/fr/sejoursoffresspeciales/mini-cure-special-aidant-la-lechere-les-bains-savoie/
Lamalou-les-Bains	https://www.chainethermale.fr/lamalou-les-bains
Néris-les-Bains	https://www.thermes-neris.com
Saint-Paul-lès-Dax	https://www.lesthermesdax.fr/?gclid=Cj0KCQjwjPaCBhDkARIsAISZN7STI28P2XcL4REjDAb7wvOwaytbJKOjGjG-PYnr5HGceF3E1cpb2hIaAqAIEALw_wcB
Saujon	https://www.thermes-saujon.fr/cure-thermale/
Thalassotherapy Center	
Hendaye	https://www.thalassoblanco.com/fr/thalasso/les-cures-thalasso/sejours-4-a-6-jours/sejours-zenitude/cure-cocooning-speciale-aidant-cure-cocooning-speciale-aidant/

Table 5.1. *Corpus of Internet pages of thermal and thalassotherapy establishments devoted to short-term thermal care for family caregivers*

The second study analyzes the point of view of seven actors of the thermal sector (see Table 5.3) through in-depth interviews carried out face to face or remotely between March 2021 and May 2021 of a duration varying between 45 minutes and one hour and a half.

Themes	Subtopics
Content analysis of web pages dedicated to short-term thermal care for caregivers	Is it easy to find the web page(s) dedicated to the short-term thermal care for caregivers on the establishment's website? How is the information on the short-term thermal care for caregivers organized on the website (number of pages, product sheets, listings)? What information is given about the short-term thermal care for caregivers (services offered, price, duration)? What are the conditions of access to the short-term thermal care for caregivers (reservation, capacity, dates)?
Analysis of discourse types	This analysis looks at the existence and content of the different discourses used: informational discourse (vocabulary relating to health, vocabulary referring to family caregivers); commercial discourse (marketing vocabulary; seductive vocabulary) and the degree of precision on the intended target (evocation of the target, width of this target, definition).
Analysis of layout quality	This analysis is based on the study of colors (use, number), visuals (use, number) and the general design of the web page(s) dedicated to the short-term thermal care for caregivers on the institution's website (highlighting of words, variation in font size, organization of spaces, text management).
URL referencing analysis	This study concerns the web page(s) referenced via the online tool Outiref.fr.

Table 5.2. *List of criteria for website content analysis*

This research combines the study of online content and the logic of actors in order to improve understanding of the spa's commercial strategy and the content of the offer proposed to the caregiver. More generally, the aim is to complete the limited knowledge on the online communication supports offered to caregivers (Atifi and Gaglio 2012).

In a first part, the figure of the caregiver in the thermal offer will be highlighted, questioning the adaptation of this last one to the targeted public. In a second part, this strategy of seduction will be approached through the particularities of the work of communication of the thermal establishments near this target.

Structure	Role in the structure	Interview reference
Thermal establishment	Director/ Head of the Health Prevention Division	Interview 1
Thermal establishment	Head of the Health Division	Interview 2
Thermal establishment	Director	Interview 3
Thermal establishment	Marketing and Communication Manager	Interview 4
Online platform for booking spa treatments	Marketing Assistant	Interview 5
Travel agency specializing in caregivers	Customer and Service Provider Manager	Interview 6
Company providing services in the spa sector	Independent Operator	Interview 7

Table 5.3. *Sample of interviewees*

5.2. The question of adapting the spa offer to a specific audience

5.2.1. *The caregiver: a legitimate target for the spa industry*

While in 1986, the World Health Organization recognized the scientific validity of thermal medicine, from the beginning of the 1990s, the needs and the habits of the French population evolved. With the development of tourism, populations abandoned thermalism which did not stop declining until the middle of the 2000s generating an 18% global loss in frequentation (Conseil national du tourisme, section des politiques territoriales et du développement durable, 2011[3]; Sonnet and Lestrelin 2017). Many spas were abandoned and then closed, victims of an aging image (linked to outdated equipment and practices) and skepticism about the effectiveness of cures. The resorts were sold to large groups who wanted to revive the spa

---

3 Conseil national du tourisme, section des politiques territoriales et du développement durable (2011), "La diversification des activités des stations thermales", chaired by P. Moisset, Ministère de l'Économie, des Finances et de l'Industrie, p. 13.

economy (La Chaîne Thermale du Soleil, ValVital, EuroThermes, France Thermes, for example).

This thermalism crisis paved the way to a marketing repositioning (Penez 2004; Jennings 2014; Roques and Bouvier 2018) leading to a new commercial offer. Beyond a better sanitary organization of care, the positioning is now centered on fitness by valuing balneotherapy and the thermo-ludique. The image of well-being is added to that of traditional treatments. Some resorts are modernizing, placing preventive healthcare at the heart of the spa stay and moving towards offers similar in title to those offered by thalassotherapy centers. In addition to the installation of new technologies for modernized treatments (sprinklers, steamers, integral mud baths, blood stimulating water corridors), the strategies and techniques of promotion and communication are improving.

The conquest of new clientele is the result of a refined marketing segmentation: young seniors, on the one hand, to renew the clientele of the 18-day cures and, on the other hand, active people suffering from psychosomatic, chronic physical pathologies for short-term thermal care (2–12 days). Special programs of non-conventional cures, redesigned both in terms of care and additional activities, have been created to take care of ourselves and relieve certain ailments (leg problems, back pain, anti-stress, all-inclusive package for caregivers, etc.). It is well within this offer of short-term thermal care that the one dedicated to caregivers finds its place.

The evolution of thermalism, via these unconventional short-term thermal care which have become complementary to the conventional cures, is unanimously recognized ("We realize that in the field of thermalism, we have to reinvent ourselves," interview 4; "The thermal baths are trying to develop. It is a general reflection that they lead," interview 5). It follows the loss of attractiveness of the thermal baths reinforced by the current sanitary situation ("the thermal establishment is today in a complicated situation. Its image is aging", interview 5).

These short stays are aimed at a clientele (either as a complement to a conventional cure, or experiencing aches and pains or a need for relaxation) who cannot spare three weeks or, more recently, at people who support patients or assist family members suffering from long-term illnesses on a day-to-day basis: family caregivers. This clientele, sometimes already acquired, has new constraints that turn them away from the conventional cure ("the clientele who used to do three-week cures and who now can no longer do so because one person in the couple has become frail has switched to this type of cure", interview 6). The caregivers also lack availability but the profile is well established ("the people who care come from the family circle (spouses, children). Sometimes the children care for their parents", interview 4; "There are two types of caregivers: caregivers who provide motor assistance and who need muscle relaxation and psychological caregivers who have psychological overload", interview 4).

The caregivers are part of a target recently explored (2/3 years) by seven thermal establishments in France and one thalassotherapy center following the observation of the absence of a dedicated offer ("The thermal baths already welcome the patient but must also be able to welcome the carer and to answer to their needs", interview 1; "an internal observation because the thermal baths welcome several patients, and their caregivers accompany them without taking advantage of a cure", interview 2). This target is identified by these establishments following the regular contact they have with it via the therapy client it cares for ("they are legitimate in proposing a cure for caregivers because they are in contact with them every day", "the spa is legitimate regarding a cure for caregivers because it can answer everything", interview 7).

The commercial offer formulated for this target group of caregivers is still in the process of emerging, which means that it is still largely confidential, including for the caregivers themselves. "The caregiver cure is not the product we think of. We think more about the psychological label" (interview 7). To sum up, if "while thermalism has a role to play in this public health problem" (interview 1), "thalassotherapy center has all the right tools. It has the right environment, it is not too medicalized" (interview 2). We understood the following clearly: to develop a short-term thermal care for the caregivers is a task that is still in progress but with a real stake for the survival of thermalism. This is where there is a necessity to give a very particular importance to the proposed offer.

5.2.2. *Short-term thermal care for caregivers in search of differentiating content*

Some thermal or thalassotherapy establishments are developing an offer for family caregivers with a certain freedom of content. This is attributable to the absence of a formal health framework for non-contracted cures in general ("For the non-medical thermal care cure, there is no protocol. It is shorter but totally financed by the patient. So the approach is different", interview 7). The carer interested in the dedicated short-term thermal care may thus find it difficult to find their way around.

Indeed, the designation of short-term thermal care for caregivers is not identical in all establishments ("cocooning cure for caregivers" in the thalassotherapy center; "caregiver module", "respite for caregivers", "stay for caregivers" in the thermal establishments). This offer is based on the promise of providing simple moments of letting go and its content is always based on thermal treatments (mud applications, body massages, thermal water showers) or marine treatments (in the case of thalassotherapy) and non-thermal treatments more or less adapted to the non-professional caregiver (relaxation sessions, conferences on the subject, meditation workshops, appointments with professionals (dietitian, nurse, sophrologist) for 100% of the cases studied).

Today, the thermal offer proposed to the carer is summarized to a "standardized offer [...]. We are going to find in one what we find in the other (swimming pool, mud, etc.)", interview 7) what questions on its specificity ("the thermal establishments offer a bath, swimming pool, mud. This goes with everything finally if we don't accompany it with a specific form of care", interview 5). To this day, is the degree of adaptation sufficient? "The thermal spas only add modules not taken into account by Social Security" (interview 5), and this stay has difficulty in differentiating itself from a mini prevention cure ("the thermal cure for caregivers is a mini prevention-health cure according to the thermal establishment even if the brand changes", interview 6). Besides, some spas, which do not have short-term thermal care for caregivers, welcome these last ones in programs oriented towards prevention-health.

The short-term thermal care offered to family caregivers is more homogeneous in terms of their duration: six out of eight places offer this combination of five to six days of care and workshops, one includes it as a complementary option to a conventional 18-day cure and one establishment offers this time on a single day (during National Caregivers' Day).

Concerning the prices of the proposed services, there are many offers. A single day costs €30 and can cost up to €1,374 for six days in a thalassotherapy center. Optional offers ranging from €90 to €150 are proposed in addition to an 18-day conventional cure, which is not easily compatible with a caregiver situation. Some "all-inclusive" week offers ranging from €197 to €500 in a thermal establishment are thus offered to the carer. The short-term thermal care for caregivers is considered as a product of appeal and is part of a strategy of price penetration for the thermal establishment. The aim of the short-term thermal care is strategic, finding its place in the vast movement of repositioning of the thermal establishment mentioned above. "We pull the price down, the main goal is to conquer new customers, who come first of all for a six day cure and who, after having experienced the cure, will surely come back for another three weeks", (interview 4). On the other hand, thalassotherapy centers want to "offer an up-market, more powerful treatment" (interview 5).

As far as access conditions are concerned, this type of cure only works on reservation (100% of the cases), notably because of the specificity of the planned workshops. Thus, while some allow reservations throughout the year, others (and this is generally the case for thermal establishments that operate by sessions) offer one or two periods of specific short-term thermal care for caregivers during the year, as for any other type of fitness program of this type (fibromyalgia, etc.). All registrations are made with the establishments concerned, which will provide the necessary information (course, period, rates, etc.). This also requires the training of customer service personnel for this type of service. Few establishments communicate on their websites the number of places available for these sessions. The information should probably be given when the caregiver registers for the treatment. For the one that does provide this information (the Saujon spa), the groups of caregivers are generally of 12–14 people maximum.

While some establishments easily reveal the programs and detail them, others only provide information on the dates of the short-term thermal care and the price with a non-exhaustive list of possible treatments to be carried out. The offers proposed to caregivers are not very well developed for some of them and vary in terms of duration, price and services included. There is no common scheme between them, and this can discourage the target public from receiving a treatment.

Elaborating short-term thermal care for caregivers is all the more difficult as the spa sector is confronted with problems already underlined by academic research works: the grouping under the designation of "caregiver", of people with different profiles, expectations and personal situations (Pennec 1999) as well as the variety of needs linked to the caregiver's situation (well-being, training in the support of the assisted person and, possibly, administrative help). While the need for a "multiform and better adjusted offer" (Kenigsberg et al. 2013) of respite approaches has already been underlined, the question of the degree of adaptation of the commercial offer comes up against the dilemma opposing hypersegmentation and marketing counter-segmentation and more generally, the problem of the commercial niche that is interesting but can prove dangerous for the finances of the spa if the number of participants is insufficient.

We will study now, in more detail, the communication of the thermal establishments towards the target of the caregivers.

5.3. The seduction strategy of caregivers in question

5.3.1. *The informational approach to communication is preferred*

Online requests for information about family caregivers have increased dramatically since 2004, as shown in the curve in Figure 5.1.

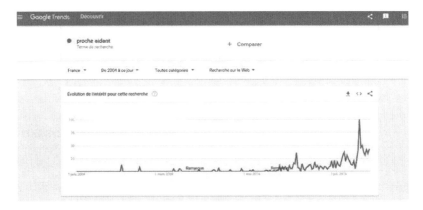

Figure 5.1. *Status of online searches by Internet users using the words "proche aidant", French for caregiver, source Google Trends, accessed on May 14, 2021*

Most of the sites consulted that mention the French for caregiver, and are therefore the best referenced naturally on search engines, refer to press articles, discussion forums and sites of associations for family caregivers that aim to support them in their daily tasks. This means that a caregiver consults sites more to get information and share their experience than to take some time for themselves and to breathe[4]. When caregivers search the Internet, they want to obtain medical information as well as practical information, support and exchange on the topic (Dubreuil and Hazif-Thomas 2013). In short, the discourse addressed to caregivers, on websites in particular, from associations of family caregivers or lucrative organizations, follows an informational

---

4 According to the Ipsos/Macif 2020 survey, 62% of the caregivers questioned felt a state of intense exhaustion and 74% said they needed a break to breathe.

logic (Romeyer 2018). Yet, the actors in the second category are initiating a more marketing approach (Chauzal-Larguier and Rouquette 2017).

On the other hand, no information is available about the search on the Web for the terms "wellness spa caregivers", "caregiver thermal baths", "caregiver thermal care" and "caregiver rest"[5]. This first observation confirms a fact ("there is no demand about the cure for caregivers. This subject did not give rise to any request for information or feedback" (interview 5). This lack of interest on the part of the caregivers for specialized sites related to the spa can be explained by at least two reasons: the difficulty in identifying oneself as a caregiver (Charlier 2018) and the lack of knowledge about this short-term thermal care among the caregivers themselves. "If information about the caregiver cure does not reach the caregiver, he or she may miss out". However, the Internet is one of the preferred media for getting information from home ("the advantage of presenting caregiver cures on websites is that the information is directly accessible for them", interview 5).

The information given on the sites of the various establishments is very variable. The size of the information found on each site is also heterogeneous, ranging from a few lines without any photograph to a complete Internet page with a downloadable sheet on this same page giving the information in detail (or included in a thermal guide of the establishment which devotes half a page or a page to it). It is therefore quite difficult for the caregiver, who has not yet decided on the choice of an establishment, to make a comparison at this stage.

Concerning the form, 100% of the studied places (thermal baths and thalassotherapy) use an informational discourse coming from the lexical field of health and the therapeutic approach ("caregivers", "physical and psychological fatigue", "dependence", "disability"), as underlined in Table 5.4 with an even stronger representation on the websites of thermal establishments.

---

5 In English: helping cure, caregiver thermal baths, caregiver and caregiver rest.

Words very present in the informational discourse	
"Caregivers", "physical and psychological fatigue", "dependence", "disability", "care", "cure", "isolated people"…	
Seduction discourse of the thermal establishments	**Seduction discourse of the thalassotherapy center**
"take a step back", "escape the guilt", "well-being", "let go", "second wind", "time to pause"…	"our hosts", "cancellation conditions", "cocooning", "zenitude", "take care of yourself", "don't wait to crack"…

Table 5.4. *Summary of the content of the thermal establishments' websites*

On the other hand, the commercial discourse, which by definition is meant to be reassuring and seductive, is more frequent on the website of the thalassotherapy establishment studied ("cocooning", "zenitude"). In this case, it is accompanied by a multitude of services (booking button, information and callback requests, contact form). This type of discourse is also used, but to a lesser extent, by the thermal establishments where the services are not put forward.

The choice of words also differs; thalassotherapy seems to be positioned more on the prevention niche ("take care of yourself", "don't wait to crack"), whereas the thermal establishment is more attached to a more curative dimension of the affection where the short-term thermal care is presented as a parenthesis to regain strength ("time to pause") before plunging back into the daily life. Is this useful or even sufficient to encourage people to subscribe to this offer?

The presentation of the services (quality of the layout, especially the colors, photos, design) is different from one site to another. The common point of all these pages is the use of blue and turquoise colors to present the offer because it reminds of water and generally determines the color used for thermalism. The rest of the presentation is often quite changeable. Some establishments illustrate their information page with a photograph of a treatment, others do not. The size of the explanation varies from a quarter page to a quadruple page with a full page. The titles and blocks are mostly not highlighted, except in the case of the thalassotherapy treatment. The colors used by the sites of the thermal establishments are often different from the graphic charters of the thermal companies and can seem little thought (example of the mixture of blue, turquoise, purple, yellow for the offer of Bagnères-de-Bigorre).

From a general point of view, the presentations of the short-term thermal care for caregivers presented on the sites of thermal establishments are less worked, without respected graphic charter, sometimes written in black and very sober where only the price is highlighted. The aim here is to give information, sometimes incomplete and not updated, without exploiting it to create desire.

On the contrary, in the case of thalassotherapy, the page is neater. The blocks are distinct and clear to facilitate the search for the headings, which makes the caregiver want to find out more. They are also encouraged to register and helped to do so ("receive a call back for more information").

With this stay for caregivers, the spa sector does not reach its goal. It does not succeed, indeed, in detaching itself from its original positioning.

> French thermalism has an image of treatment of diseases. It is connoted health, curative. We don't go there for prevention. That's why we go for thalassotherapy, with a clear mind. If you go to a spa, it's because you're sick (interview 5).

However, because they do not recognize themselves as such, caregivers largely underestimate their need for help (Mollard 2009; Brülhart et al. 2013; Pierron-Robinet et al. 2018) and it remains difficult to formulate their needs (Amieva et al. 2012). Hence, the question of the relevance for the thermal establishment to remain on an informational and curative positioning that may not touch the caregiver, for lack of projection of a person in this role?

5.3.2. *Good referencing of the websites of thermal establishments is poorly exploited*

Generally speaking, the referencing of the websites of the thermal establishments is well constructed, contrary to that of the thalassotherapy center. The information searched for on search engines is very easy to find in most cases with the simple keywords "cure aidant + nom de la station" (treatment cure + resort name). In general, the first three results are good. In the case of the spa resorts of the "chaîne thermale du soleil" group, the information is to be found again on the group's website, which groups together the different sites of the resorts (global communication to all).

This good result can be explained in part by the fact that these sites are often consulted first because they represent a safe value for patients. Indeed, thermal establishments benefit from an image as "historic players" in water treatment, whose expertise is recognized by the World Health Organization, and from a certain notoriety among the general public.

For the thermal establishments, the choice of the title is often short but well-chosen with good meta-descriptions from the point of view of the number but mainly by keywords which do not really correspond to the target of "caregivers": they remain mainly centered around the terms "cure", "thermal" and "rest". It is then possible that these few pages (or half-pages) are drowned in the website of the structures (conventional cures and short-term thermal care included) and that it is this set that generates a better global referencing. This is explained by the following reason:

> concerning the purchase of keywords concerning Google referencing, the thermal establishment is not going to buy "non-medical thermal care" or "short-term thermal care" but rather rheumatology cures for example (interview 7).

In the end, we can say that the websites of the studied thermal establishments have common characteristics and combine a well-constructed referencing with the content of websites little worked as well on the content as on the form. The difference is made with the private thalassotherapy site which uses employs truer marketing around the caregiver as well in the content as in the form but which does not have the same strength of referencing on the Web. The thermal establishments do not manage to take advantage of this good referencing because of the lack of a convincing approach of their communication on the Internet. Even more seriously, the thermal sector does not succeed with the short-term thermal care helping to promote the new positioning, lighter and more focused on well-being, that it wants to set up from the non-medical thermal care.

Such observations question the degree of involvement of the thermal establishment towards this young target and on its desire to implement a real marketing strategy allowing it to reposition itself by including this new market segment. In the field, the answer is unanimous: the non-reimbursed cure is the way found by thermalism to ensure its economic perenniality ("The discourse on non-reimbursed cures is a marketing discourse", interview 5; "It's unfortunate, it's marketing", interview 4). The commercial dimension given to the discourse here is visible ("The thermal establishment is going to communicate on its non-medical thermal care in a more commercial way than for the conventional cure", interview 7). Hence, the obvious interest to compose an offer at a lower cost by drawing from the existing treatments. Numerous targets, including caregivers, are envisaged and sometimes this leads to the implementation of a specific short-term thermal care. The caregiver is seen as just another commercial target. "Yes, the caregiver is a marketing target" (interview 1).

Wanting to conquer this target is not easy. While the non-professional carer is today well identified by thermalism as by thalassotherapy, he remains poorly recognized and the risk of involuntary stigmatization through the proposed offer is not to be excluded. Indeed, "to offer a product to a particular target is always dangerous. It can give a dangerous image. It can be very badly perceived because caregivers are suffering people" (interview 2).

However, the short-term thermal care for caregivers is not devoid of assets that can be promoted commercially, as is the case on certain online platforms: "this type of stay allows caregivers to breathe and avoid physical and psychological fatigue. The 'caregivers' spa cure is a real moment between the patients who meet around a common point"[6]. Moreover, it finds its public when it tries ("the return is

---

6 See: www.lescuristes.fr.

good", interview 6). However, with an assistant who is not very available and for lack of attractive, up-to-date and clear communication, it does not always lead to sufficient demand being generated. Hence, the decision of some thermal establishments not to maintain this short-term thermal care in their offer in the future[7].

The caregivers, as all of those who visit the thermal baths within the framework of a non-medical thermal care, change the practices of spa clients and can make the image of the resorts change, which see the opportunity to reinvent themselves and to open to these multiple types of stays. More widely, it is part of a desire to conquer a younger clientele which would perhaps never have turned to thermalism ("So that a cure is said to be fully efficient, it is necessary to offer three years of cures, and the benefit of the cures is supposed to last longer and longer after each year", interview 4) and that it will be necessary to build loyalty ("Today, we have to get out of the conventional 18-day cures and offer a shorter program, 6 or 12 days, keeping in mind that all these programs are the means to conquer tomorrow's clientele (caregivers, those with Parkinson's, Alzheimer's, Covid) this year", interview 4). Hence, the need to "conduct a reflection at all levels of communication" (interview 5) by associating other actors (associations, doctors). The role of the attending physician is not to be neglected because this one is already identified ("They come following the advice of the doctors members of the CNET (French National Council of the Thermal Establishments) who promote the cure to the doctors. They have worked on the prescription of thermal cures with the doctors", interview 4).

5.4. Conclusion

The research work offers three kinds of contributions. This communication proposes a first inventory of the commercial offer intended for the caregivers in thermal establishments. Besides a measure of the interest given to this target, this research work allows a

---

7 Two spas did not offer this short-term thermal care in 2021. They were therefore not included in our comparative analysis of websites and not counted in the statistics of this research work.

comparative analysis of the content of the proposed offer by questioning the degree of adaptation to the caregiver and to the offering establishment. Secondly, the comparative analysis underlines the progress of thermal establishments in the setting up of a commercial offer intended for the carer. Thirdly, at a more theoretical level, this marketing path of the thermal establishment questions about the conditions and the content of a marketing of the carer and about its possible integration in a more general marketing strategy developed by the thermal establishment.

We can question the real role of establishments offering a cure for caregivers. Indeed, it is undeniable that through this commercial target, they develop a new marketing strategy facilitating, as we have said, a repositioning that contributes to their survival. However, it seems relevant to question the other contributions of this treatment, going beyond the sole marketing framework studied in this chapter. Firstly, on the potential social innovation[8] that is engaged with this cure. Secondly, the role of the thermal and thalassotherapy establishment towards the caregivers joins the one recognized to the health professionals, i.e. "not only to relieve physical pain, but to take into consideration the moral suffering" (Berti 2017, p. 26).

The perception of this treatment should be studied by questioning the caregivers themselves, as well as the actors who can give an informed opinion on the relevance of this commercial offer: medical personnel (doctor, psychologist, etc.) and the network of actors around the caregiver (associations, communal and intercommunal social action centers, local information and coordination centers, etc.).

---

8 For the Social Innovation Working Group of the *Conseil Supérieur de l'Economie Sociale et Solidaire*, "social innovation consists of developing new responses to new or poorly satisfied social needs under the current conditions of the market and social policies, by involving the participation and cooperation of the actors concerned, in particular users. These innovations concern the product or service, as well as the mode of organization and distribution, in areas such as aging, early childhood, housing, health, the fight against poverty, exclusion, discrimination, etc.".

5.5. References

Amieva, H., Rullier, L., Bouisson, J., Dartigues, F., Dubois, O., Salamon, R. (2012). Attentes et besoins des aidants de personnes souffrant de maladie d'Alzheimer. *Revue d'épidémiologie et de santé publique*, 60(3), 231–238.

Atifi, H. and Gaglio, G. (2012). L'Internet des aidants. In *Internet et santé : acteurs, usages et appropriations*, Levy, J.J. and Thoër, C. (eds). Presses de l'Université du Québec, Quebec.

Balcou-Debussche, M. (2006). *L'éducation des malades chroniques, une approche ethnosociologique*. Archives Contemporaines Éditions, Paris.

Belorgey, N., Pinsard, E., Rousseau, J. (2016). Naissance de l'aidant. Les pratiques des employeurs face à leurs salariés soutenant un proche. *Genèses*, 1(102), 67–88.

Berti, E. (2017). *Une présence idéale*. Flammarion, Paris.

Bloch, M.-A. (2012). Les aidants et l'émergence d'un nouveau champ de recherche interdisciplinaire. *Vie sociale*, 4(4), 11–29.

Brülhart, D., Brügger, S., Sottas, B. (2013). Les proches aidants ont aussi besoin d'aide. *Revue internationale de soins palliatifs*, 28(3), 193–196.

Caradec, V. (2009). Vieillir, un fardeau pour les proches ? *Lien social et politiques*, 62, 111–122.

Chanial, P. and Gaglio, G. (2013). Aidons les aidants. Une initiative mutualiste face au marché de la dépendance. *Revue du Mauss*, 41, 121–139.

Charlap, C., Caradec, V., Chamahian, A., Kushtanina, V. (2019). Être salarié et aider une proche âgé dépendant : droits sociaux et arrangements locaux. *Revue française des affaires sociales*, 1, 181–198.

Charlier, E. (2018). Aidants proches : une reconnaissance en demi-teinte ? *La Revue nouvelle*, 4(4), 59–64.

Chauzal-Larguier, C. and Rouquette, S. (2017). Médias sociaux et associations d'aidants familiaux. Risques ou opportunités ? *Les cahiers du numérique*, 13(2), 75–104.

Desfour, H. (2011). Actualisation sur les actions d'éducation déjà en place en milieu thermal. *La presse thermale et climatique*, 13–20.

Domingo, P. and Verite, C. (2011). Aider un parent dépendant : comment concilier vies familiale, sociale et professionnelle ? *Politiques sociales et familiales*, 105(1), 31–46.

Dubreuil, A. and Hazif-Thomas, C. (2013). Les aidants et la santé sur Internet ou les aidantsnautes s'entraident. *Neurologie/Psychiatrie/ Gériatrie*, 13, 250–255.

Gagnon, M., Beaudry, C., Boies, J. (2018). L'amélioration des conditions de travail des aidants par le prisme de la conciliation des temps sociaux : vecteur d'un meilleur climat organisationnel et de la rétention des employés. *Ad Machina*, 2(1), 19–34.

Husson, G.-P. (1996). Historique du thermalisme en France. *Cahiers de l'Association scientifique européenne pour l'eau et la santé*, 1, 3–6.

Jazé-Charvolin, M.-R. (2014). Les stations thermales : de l'abandon à la renaissance. Une brève histoire du thermalisme en France depuis l'Antiquité. *In Situ, Revue des patrimoines*, 24, 1–15.

Jennings, E.T. (2014). Donneuses d'eau. Une profession au cœur du thermalisme français (1840–1914). *Sociétés & Représentations*, 2(38), 143–170.

Kenigsberg, P.-A., Ngatcha-Robert, L., Villez, M., Gzil, F., Berard, A., Fremontier, M. (2013). Le répit : des réponses pour les personnes atteintes de la maladie d'Alzheimer ou de maladies apparentées et leurs aidants – Évolutions de 2000 à 2011. *Recherches familiales*, 1(10), 57–69.

Le Bihan-Youinou, B. and Martin, C. (2006). Travailler et prendre soin d'un parent âgé dépendant. *Revue Travail, genre et sociétés*, 16(2), 77–96.

Lohez, M. (2000). Thermalisme et tourisme : les évolutions récentes en France. *L'information géographique*, 4, 314–321.

Martin, C. (2010). Concilier vie familiale et vie professionnelle : un objectif européen dans le modèle français des politiques de la famille ? *Informations sociales*, 1(157), 114–123.

Miles, B.M. and Huberman, A.M. (2003). *Analyse des données qualitatives*. De Boeck, Brussels.

Mollard, J. (2009). Aider les proches. *Gérontologie et société*, 32(1–2), 257–272.

Nabeth, M. (2019). La santé, les aidants et la micro-assurance. *Banque & stratégie*, 385, 6–12.

Pailhé, A. and Solaz, A. (2009). *Entre famille et travail : des arrangements de couple aux pratiques des employeurs*. La Découverte, Paris.

Penez, J. (2004), *Histoire du thermalisme en France au XIXème siècle*. Economica, Paris.

Pennec, S. (1999). Les aidants : déconstruire une catégorisation sociale par trop généraliste. *Gérontologie et société*, 6(89), 41–61.

Piazzon, F. (2018). *Absentéisme : l'alerte rouge. Penser et repenser le Travail*. Débats Publics, Paris.

Pierron-Robinet, G., Bonnet, M., Mariage, A., Puyraveau, M. (2018). Les incidences du sentiment de culpabilité sur la demande d'aide de l'aidant familial. *Annales Médico-Psychologiques*, 176(2), 170–176.

Romeyer, H. (2018). TIC et santé : entre information médicale et information de santé. *TIC & Société*, 2(1), 27–44.

Roques, C. and Bouvier, C.-E. (2018). Prévention en médecine thermale. In *La médecine thermale, données scientifiques*, Queneau, P. and Roques, C. (eds). John Libbey Eurotext, Montrouge.

Rouquette, S. (2009). *L'analyse des sites internet*. De Boeck, Louvain.

Sonnet, A. and Lestrelin, L. (2017). Thermalisme : la montée en puissance du bien-être. *Jurisport*, 173, 42–45.

Toulier, B. (2004). Les réseaux de la villégiature en France. *In Situ, Revue des patrimoines*, 4, 1–24.

Weisz, G. (2002). Le thermalisme en France au XXe siècle. *Médecines/ Sciences*, 18(1), 101–108.

PART 2

Narrative Medicine and
Patient and Caregiver Hermeneutics

6

When the Doctor Becomes a Patient: The Relationship Between the Caregiver and the Breast Cancer Patient in *Demain nous appartient*

This article explores how the French series, *Demain nous appartient,* broadcast daily by TF1 since 2017, depicts one of its protagonists facing breast cancer. In this narrative broadcast in 2019, the particularity of the character is to be both doctor and patient. This dual position allows the scriptwriters to show the care pathway for a patient, to convey messages of prevention, to recall patient rights. By opting for a story of the disease rooted in narrative medicine and the emotional journey of the patient, the series offers a polyphonic narration featuring the patient, the caregiver or caregivers and their family circle to which viewers can easily relate.

6.1. Introduction

Since July 17, 2017, *Demain nous appartient*, a French soap opera, has been airing daily in prime time access Monday through Friday on TF1. In this ensemble show and family series, the hospital is at the heart of many storylines, with some recurring characters in the series being doctors within a hospital institution.

Chapter written by Laurence CORROY and Emilie ROCHE.

Several narrative arcs are intertwined within each episode, with different temporalities of interweaving storylines and denouement, resuming a scenaristic system previously observed in *Plus belle la vie*[1]. Generally, three temporalities confront each other, linked to the genres used: a purely comic plot which is developed then resolved during the episode, a tragicomic plot which extends over several episodes and finally a plot which unfolds over 15 or 20 episodes, i.e. three to four weeks of broadcasting, which includes a police-type mystery to be solved. The chosen story arc belongs to the third category, but, in an original way, it is not a police mystery. The plot centers on the difficulty of the director of the general medicine department of a hospital herself becoming a patient due to a serious illness, breast cancer.

During this situation of personal crisis, the doctor's medicine narrative, someone who has become a patient, who recounts and evokes doubts and fears, while having expert knowledge, will be intertwined. We will see that the medical knowledge available to the character does not spare her from the doubts and problems of a suffering body.

This narrative arc allows for a better understanding of the representations of a long illness within popular fiction as evoked by the patient, whose emotional manifestations are put into words and images, as well as of the relationship between the caregiver and the patient.

By moving in the direction of educating viewers through entertainment in which they are emotionally invested[2], the series, written by a group of writers, can possibly, through one of the series' main characters, offer a range of prevention messages that emerge based on the protagonists portrayed in three different roles, namely the patient, the doctor and the caregiver.

---

1 See Corroy, L. (2010). Un feuilleton hexagonal qui plaît : *Plus belle la vie*. In *Les jeunes et les médias, les raisons du succès*, Corroy, L. (ed.), Paris, Vuibert, Paris, 83–103.

2 On the subject of studies that have worked on the alliance of education and entertainment, see Barthes, S. (2016). Panique à la télé: La résistance bactérienne vue par les séries télévisées. *Questions de communication*, 29, 112.

Our method was to take the entire corpus, all episodes that aired between January 4, 2019 and February 19, 2019, from episode 371 to 409. This is a longer narrative arc than the average long storyline. This is due to the scriptural necessity of making a storyline about a disease known for its slow treatment. Not all the episodes aired during this period refer to it, far from it. However, when the subject is approached in an episode, several scenes are devoted to it. This allows the scriptwriters to advance the plot while allowing an ensemble positioning on the subject, featuring the patient, the caregiver(s) and the family circle. We took into account all the dialogues explicitly dedicated to Marianne Delcourt's illness, whether she appears in the scene or not. When she appears, the fact that she is a doctor and a patient offers several sequences of narrative medicine where her medical knowledge and her emotions as a patient are intertwined, without the former actually helping the latter. Knowing all the implications of the disease and the possible side-effects of the treatments is not very helpful when the character is suffering.

6.2. Narrative of the disease

Defined by Rita Charon (2015, p. 13), narrative medicine is akin to a skill that allows for intellectual and emotional consideration of the illness narrative as narrated and described by the patient. Narrative allows for the understanding and actualization of a narrative of illness in a process based on listening to, understanding the patient, which should lead to medicine as it should always be: honest, human and authentic, where the doctor–patient relationship becomes a therapeutic relationship (Charon 2015).

Emphasizing empathy for the patient also helps doctors develop an increased reflexivity for their profession (Goupy and Le Jeunne 2016). However, in the patient's medical journey as portrayed in the series, the doctor–patient relationship is not very present and the representation of the oncologist who takes charge of the patient shows a medical profession that has not integrated narrative medicine into its practices. We can see both a criticism of the system of emotional and psychological care of patients with serious illnesses as well as the choice of the scriptwriters to highlight a part of narrative medicine that relies on the patient's family circle.

In the educational guide developed by the WHO concerning patient safety, a section dedicated to communication recalls the importance of interactions with the patient and their relatives, in particular by understanding the family dynamics at work, by involving the relatives concerned so that they can eventually participate in decision-making, and by respecting the role of families in the care of the patient (WHO 2011, p. 69). In the same vein, the *Conseil de l'ordre national des médecins* (French Council of the National Order of Physicians) insists that, if the patient so wishes, they "must be able to designate a trusted person (a parent or close relative), who will support them in their steps and attend medical interviews in order to help them in their decisions" (CNOM 2011, p. 14). In fiction, narrative medicine can make it possible to show a plurality of points of view, and especially to integrate the caregiver's point of view. It is therefore not a question of a dyad but of a triad that triangulates the disease and its impact on the life of the patient and their loved ones, as well as the reverse effect of the attitude of the loved ones and the doctor on the evolution of the disease. The series gives a large place to the figure of the caregiver while allowing the patient's story of her illness to take shape. As Hélène Marche has defined it,

> the narratives of the illness are articulated around the issue of the reconstruction of a biographical crisis. In the perspective of a "narrative identity" outlined by Paul Ricoeur (1983), the narrative could thus be considered as the vector of a restructuring of subjectivity by means of forms of projections and identifications, which would make it possible to restore a continuity of the self (Marche 2020, p. 187).

It is indeed a biographical crisis that Marianne Delcourt's character is going through and her life path, as a patient, is shown to us.

In the series, the narrative of the illness is also embodied in non-verbal actions (sadness, withdrawal, crying, laughter, aggressiveness) which "can be considered as forms of narrative in the sense that they give to those who receive them narratives of the experience of the illness" (Marche 2020, p. 189). In the different episodes, the patient's emotions appear as a social language.

From shame to modesty, from the dispossession of self to
the reappropriation of one's body and life, from parading
to exhibition, the limits of the relationship to self and
others, but also the limits of biomedical power to contain
the patient's entire experience (Marche 2020, p. 188).

Research on breast cancer has also shown that the medical
profession often invites the patient to adopt a posture of struggle,
between optimism and a warrior posture in order to fight the cancer.
However, the question of the suffering that invades the body resists
language, especially medical language. The scriptwriters of *Demain
nous appartient* have chosen to deconstruct these stereotypes of the
ideal patient and the series helps to fight against the stereotypical
representations of the patient as a victim or a hero. Marianne Delcourt is
first and foremost a woman whose specificity is certainly to be both a
patient and a doctor, which does not exempt her from suffering.

6.3. Emotional journey of the patient physician

The specificity of the chosen narrative arc is linked to the patient's
professional status, who also works as a department head in a hospital.
Sandra Bonneaudeau collected testimonies from doctors who have lived
through an experience similar to the one described in the series, and her
thesis examines the particularities of sick doctors. Are they sick like any
other? She describes an "entry" into the disease "experienced as a
shock", with doctors going through a range of emotions, including "a
phase of regression during treatment" and a "feeling of revolt in the face
of the disease" (Bonneaudeau 2011, pp. 47–48).

In her research in clinical and social psychology, Ginette
Francequin shows that breast cancer imposes a femininity to be rebuilt
in regard to the patient, whatever her journey. This is divided into
three acts: the shock of the announcement, the doubt and fear, and the
mourning for a body that has been expropriated and will no longer be
as it was before and will be transformed. In the first act, that of the
announcement of the disease, the person is confronted with a sudden
announcement that constitutes a psychological shock. A state of shock
may follow the announcement, especially since the patient is then

reminded of her own vulnerability. The announcement is also the promise of a burdensome and long treatment to which the removal of the breast(s) is often added.

> The announcement of the diagnosis is therefore a key moment, the one that makes the subject switch "from the world of the healthy to the world of the sick on borrowed time". It is the tipping point into uncertainty (Francequin 2012, p. 80).

After the shock of the diagnosis, the series shows how Dr. Marianne Delcourt experiences anxiety regarding death, which is expressed by the desire to give one of her daughters, as a testamentary act, a precious piece of jewelry, without expressing the reasons for this gift. She cries, which is quite unusual, as the ethos of the character, who has been on the air for more than a year and is well known to regular viewers of the show, is built on the fact that she has a very strong character.

In the exercise of her profession, she is not very sensitive to doubt and to the expression of a fallible self. Her ethos as a physician is repeatedly reminded and mobilized. As she becomes a patient, she reminds those around her that she is a doctor. But this ethos does not prove to be of much help in the face of the affects that overwhelm her. While we might think, as the hospital director reminds her, that she is a doctor and therefore better equipped than anyone else in this context, this is not the case. Overwhelmed by anguish, she tearfully responds that, on the contrary, she knows what awaits her, exhaustion, irascibility and weakening because, she says, "even the strongest patients have their lives disrupted" (episode 373).

Anxiety of death quickly takes the form of a lack of care, of a desire to postpone treatment in order to devote to our list of desires. In this respect, Fanny Soum-Pouyalet reminds us that "the world of cancer care is a highly emotional place, given the seriousness of the pathologies that are treated" (Soum-Pouyalet 2006), equating all forms of cancer with death in the minds of patients.

After the shock, come the doubt and the fear which are defense reflexes facing an unbearable situation. Researchers point to denial as a recurrent phase because it allows for fighting against identity and narcissistic damage. Refusal is not denial, "everything happens as if we had not seen anything", we try to eliminate an embarrassing representation on this part of the body, on this reality and what we have perceived (the breast tumor, the affected body image) (Francequin 2012, p. 45).

In the case of Marianne Delcourt, this led her to refuse care. Rebellious and angry, she decides to drink and dance. The chosen excerpt features Marianne Delcourt and the hospital director, who is in love with her:

Renaud: Er, what are you doing here?

Marianne: Well you see, I'm allowing myself a little bit of fun.

Renaud: With tomato juice?

Marianne: Bloody Mary. It reminds me of my punk nights.

Renaud: Did you go to punk parties?

Marianne: Well, of course not, but I should have.

Renaud: And as a doctor, do you think it's the best time in your life to get drunk at nap time?

Marianne: Well, it was either that or Xanax, and as an anxiolytic, I prefer alcohol.

Renaud: In small doses.

Marianne: Who cares about the dosage?

Renaud: Well listen you know what, I'll take you home, it's a better idea. Shall we go?

Marianne: Oh no, I barely had a sip of that stuff.

Renaud: Well, it's still a big sip.

Marianne: Oh yes, you're right. I need a second one. Please.

Renaud: Don't get drunk. It's really not the solution.

Marianne: Fuck you.

Renaud: Ah, classy drinking, I see.

Marianne: Fuck my cancer. Fuck the metastases. Fuck the mastectomy, fuck the radiation. And fuck everyone who tells me about it.

Renaud: I totally agree with you. Fuck all that too.

Marianne: Well, there you go. And since I'm not working today, well if I feel like lining up Bloody Marys at the hospital's service meetings, well, I'll do it.

Renaud: Well, finally, I think you may be right.

Marianne: Of course I'm right. Shall I order you one?

Renaud: And how!

Marianne: Two![3]

The director of the hospital, following this exchange, takes her home and a love affair begins. Marianne Delcourt asks him to stay, because she wants to "feel alive". The will to feel alive will be expressed by taking risks. Renting a racing car that she drives at open throttle on the highway, then taking her first scuba diving experience are the first rough patches. The character then wants to start skydiving. Her lists of desires feature so many death-defying stunts, to put herself in danger – paradoxically giving herself the impression of controlling her destiny – in order to live intensely in the present moment. Taking risks is an attempt to regain control of her life and her body by choosing the perils she faces, unlike the disease that imposes them on her.

Finally forced to accept care under the pressure of her ex-husband who threatens to tell her daughters everything, she finally complies. She then enters another phase, where she accepts her emotions and fears and expresses them. Hermeneutics of the self are then

3 Episode 372, aired on January 7, 2019, from 15 mins 10 to 16 mins 25. Place of action: a restaurant, the Spoon. Characters present in the scene: Marianne Delcourt, head of department, Renaud, director of the hospital.

constructed, which describe both the possible effects of the illness on her body and her psychological state. As she herself says, "she knows how cancer evolves" (episode 380).

The various emotions expressed by the character are quite similar to those described by subjects who have had a similar experience. While the advantages of being a doctor are mentioned – care considered better than that of non-physician patients, often linked to networks of solicited colleagues, a sharpened understanding of their illness, treatments and its consequences, capacities of self-description of their symptoms and an autonomy superior to some patients with an identical pathology – the limits, even the singular difficulties of being a patient carer are also underlined.

The fact of becoming a patient to oneself can make one extremely sensitive to the symptoms observed. Doctors mention a possible lack of objectivity, an immediate understanding of symptoms and possible risks that can lead to a "dramatization of clinical signs", an ease in obtaining information that adds to the anxiety, sometimes causing a greater anxiety than non-doctor patients. However, this does not lead to early management, quite the contrary. Overloaded schedules, possibly with professional over-investment just after the diagnosis is announced, as well as difficulties in seeking help from a third party are cited (Bonneaudeau 2011, p. 57).

In the show, the character takes the illness as a warning. "It's an eye-opener," she says. "It's a way of telling me that I'm closer to the end than the beginning[4]." With the operation to remove the tumor scheduled, the patient expresses her anxieties about a mutilated or at least damaged body, which might no longer arouse desire. With resistance at the beginning, she also ends up accepting help from her family circle.

In the third act, described by the clinical researchers, the patients "get their act together" and "make sure" to accept their treatment(s) but they also have to mourn the body that will no longer be what it was. This stage related to care and eventual recovery involves a dissociation of the body, between the biological body subjected to

4 Episode 386, airing January 25, 2019.

treatment and the lived body; it is an experience of "extreme familiarity and great ignorance" (Francequin 2012, p. 41). Breast cancer treatment is all the more of an ordeal because the patient has no choice; she must reconcile the experience of expropriation of the body by the treatments with the intimate experience of her body.

Through Marianne Delcourt's journey as a patient, viewers are provided with essential medical advice on cancer management. The series distils medical advice and vocabulary, disseminating a health education message in small steps, coming closer to the "edutainment" of some American series that feature medical storylines (Aksakal 2015). Marjolaine Boutet, in analyzing daily series broadcast in France, notes:

> Among a mass of sweet and reassuring stories that are as quickly watched as they are forgotten, we can nevertheless find some real nuggets of high quality, and it would be wrong to neglect the cultural importance of daily soap operas which, although produced on the assembly line, often deliver real political and social messages whose influence is all the greater because of the viewers' emotional attachment to the characters who embody them (Boutet 2019, p. 68).

We could add health messages to his remark. The attachment to the characters, as well as the possibility of disseminating information concerning health over the course of the episodes of a long narrative arc, makes it possible to offer advice without turning viewers off.

The focus is on prevention through screening for breast cancer, now a common disease that requires women to have regular check-ups. Several dialogues serve to alert the viewer to the importance of early detection (the oncologist explains to his patient that her tumor is at an early stage and that she was right to be screened) and the need for reactive management. As the hospital director gently reminds her, the chances of recovery are correlated with the speed of treatment (episode 377). He returns to her in another episode, when she tells him that the discussion is over and that she will not have surgery right away. He immediately becomes concerned, reminding her of the danger of the cancer spreading and metastasizing, putting her at risk of death (episode 380).

However, the patient, whoever they may be, must be recognized as a thinking and active subject. Preserving their autonomy and free will is essential even though they are dependent on their illness and the medical profession. The patient's choices must therefore be respected: the choice to be treated, to disclose or not the existence of illness to the family. In the different episodes, Marianne Delcourt asserts her ethos as a patient who maintains her free will despite her illness. Insofar as it is her cancer, it is she who decides (episode 371). As a patient, this gives her rights (episode 401), including the right to tell her condition if, when and to whom, as it is "a decision that belongs to the patient" (episode 403).

Crying, death anxiety, anger, rebellion, impatience, pessimism, dark thoughts, fears of a failing sexuality are expressed in turn, and are listened to and answered by the two caregivers.

Her journey as a sick doctor runs counter to the emotional labor pointed out by therapists who feel compelled to bury the emotions they feel about their patients in order to conform to social expectations related to their professional context (Truc et al. 2009; Hochschild 2017). Becoming ill, accepting it, is instead for doctors to meet and embrace their emotions, an emotional journey woven throughout the plot.

The doctor's willingness to let go and accept the treatment protocol and to be supported morally by two men close to her, allowed her to begin the healing process. Here again, this attitude is in line with the fieldwork observed among doctors with a serious pathology, who advise trying to "forget their profession and become patients and only patients" (Bonneaudeau 2011, p. 57).

6.4. The role of caregivers

In the French Code of Social Action and Families, the caregiver is defined by the fact that they perform domestic work free of charge for a relative in a situation of disability or dependence. Since the beginning of the 21st century, the notion of "care" has gone far beyond that of domestic care for a family member, with caregivers taking care of their loved ones (Belorgey et al. 2016, pp. 67–68). The category remains uncertain in its naming, with caregivers being considered "natural", "family" or "non-professional", depending on whether the emphasis is on traditional solidarities within families, or on the qualification of their help as opposed to that of the medical profession (Savignat 2014).

The narrative plot focuses on the role of two characters who will surround the patient and take on the role of caregivers. Marianne Delcourt, refusing to let her daughters know about it, is guided and supported by two men – the first one being her ex-husband, the second one her current partner, also a doctor. The two male characters form a duo of caregivers, complementing each other.

Although she tries to refuse their help on several occasions, they do not give her the choice and, by their constancy, reassure her. In the case of her lover, Renaud, it is the role of confidant that is appreciated, not his medical expertise. Thus, she asks him to act "as a friend", not "as a doctor", and to forget "the coat a little" (episode 377). On this occasion, the attitude of the physician caregiver is similar to the previously cited study, which notes that when a physician has a loved one confronted with illness, fear appears to be heightened, although he cannot help but interfere to a greater or lesser extent with the care (Bonneaudeau 2011, p. 84).

An episode in which Renaud asks about her medical interviews shows this emotional and medical help:

> Renaud: Anyway, you went to see Labose, that's good, that means you decided to get treated. Have you set a date for the operation? I'll come and see you.
>
> Marianne: I don't need to be held.
>
> Renaud: But what do you think? That you're going to have an operation all by yourself and then take a cab to go home, quietly?
>
> Marianne: Yes, why not?

Renaud: I will be with you before, during and after. Whether you like it or not. I'll camp out in your living room. I will make you food. I'll give you your medicine.

Marianne: If I organize myself a little, I won't need all this.

Renaud: It's a shame to have to beg you for help.

Marianne: Renaud how can I tell you? I don't want your pity, it doesn't help me.

Renaud: Get that out of your head. It's not pity.

Marianne: Okay. But you better not look at me like I'm dying, because if I look at myself like that in your eyes...

Renaud: Not a chance. For me you are the opposite[5].

He follows these appointments, performing acts of assistance, vigilance, advice and reassurance. The love and erotic side is not omitted either. Thus, alarmed by the scars she will have after her operation, Marianne Delcourt fears no longer being seductive and losing her companion. This disarray encountered by many patients is similar to a depressive state, particularly because of the metaphorical representations linked to the breasts:

> The attack on the breast, its mutilation through mammectomy, certainly raises the question of castration anxiety in women, but also allows us to identify the emergence of other anxieties, more archaic, which struggle to be contained, and which refer to other phantasmatic valences, when they do not signal the collapse of the representative system. Even if it is culturally significant, the conflict between the nourishing breast and erotic breast does not summarize the polyvalence of the breast – oral, anal, urethral, phallic, genital breast –, breast of all the partial impulses that a trauma is able to reactivate, and which sometimes serve as levels of fixations avoiding too harmful regressions (Parat 2017, p. 101).

5 Episode 386, aired Friday, January 25, 2019, 14 mins 40 to 16 mins 30.

The help of her companion in love is fundamental for the character:

> Renaud: Marianne, you are a very beautiful woman and you have no worries about your intimate future.
>
> Marianne: But I won't be the same woman.
>
> Renaud: Obviously you are not the same as when you were 20 or 30. But you are still attractive, do you realize that? No man will stop at a scar.
>
> Marianne: I'm not so sure.
>
> Renaud: I know what I'm talking about. I will always find you attractive.
>
> Marianne: You say that now but when my breast is damaged...
>
> Renaud: Marianne, you are extremely desirable and it's not just a question of plastic. It's everything you give off. Your voice, your look, your way of being. Your whole person.
>
> Marianne: Come to my place tonight, I want you to make love to me[6].

Expressing her fears clearly allows her partner to reassure her. He frankly expresses that his sexual desire is not attached to a bodily detail but rather is tied to a holistic eroticized vision of the attachment support person. On several occasions, dialogues concerning her sexual life and the fact of remaining desirable punctuate the episodes. Renaud proves to be reliable, proving to her through his desires and declarations that he is sentimentally and sexually attached to her.

This common background is that of the private sphere which no longer takes into account the social and collective experience. This regime of intimacy is also what is shown through the character of Marianne Delcourt. Once her operation is successful, while she is undergoing a rather non-invasive radiotherapy treatment, the difficulty of re-taming her body reappears. Femininity, the damaged body

---

6 Episode 389, aired on January 30, 6 mins 22 to 9 mins 10.

and sexuality are issues of the aftermath of chemotherapy and mastectomy.

The other caregiver, André, her ex-husband, is a comical and more direct character. He does not hesitate to blackmail her a little to get her to treat herself and forces her to express her emotions and fears. He plays a role of confidant, in a relationship which allows Marianne Delcourt to formulate more easily her anxieties of death to better exorcise them. He becomes the receiver of her emotions, just like the therapist and his patient. He invites her to say everything that terrifies her, which she does:

> I'm not afraid Andre I'm terrified. I'm afraid there will be complications. I'm afraid of being in pain afterwards. I'm afraid that I won't wake up […] I'm afraid that the cancer will come back, that it was useless. I'm afraid… Of the scar… I know it's a futile consideration but I can't stop thinking about it[7].

Ten episodes later, after the operation, Marianne Delcourt still expresses her fears about the side effects of radiotherapy and the risk of cancer recurrence.

The two men provide two types of support, pragmatic and symbolic. Pragmatic, when it is a question of going with her to her medical appointments, giving her medication, feeding her when she does not have the courage to eat. But it is also a question of supporting the patient morally, by changing her ideas. Her ex-husband organizes, with the complicity of her partner, a meal where Marianne must literally eat a "crab" which represents her cancer, thus marking her will to take over[8].

The optimism of the two caregivers highlights the "right" kind of care: they adopt, as caregivers, the right distance, loving with

---

7 Episode 387, airing January 26, 2019.
8 Episode 386, aired on January 25, 2019, 17 mins 58 to 18 mins 55. At Marianne's house, with Renaud, her partner and André, her ex-husband.

constancy, while maintaining a positive attitude, a sign of empathy without sympathy. The figure of the successful caregiver turns out to be the one that consecrates the gesture of support as theorized by Tanguy Chatel:

> Supporting is not guiding, even with the best intentions in the world. It is more modestly accepting the patient's highs and lows, his angers, his denials, his silences, his wanderings as much as his joys, his laughter, and eventually his serenity, without trying to redirect or abandon him (Chatel 2010, p. 88).

This attitude contrasts with that of his daughters. When they suspect that their father may have cancer, they immediately become overly dramatic. This partly explains Dr. Delcourt's choice not to reveal her illness to them. The figure of the bad caregiver or of the caregiver who cannot help is thus sketched out:

Marianne: So what was so urgent?

Anna: We'd love your advice.

Chloe: We think Dad is sick.

Marianne: Really?

Chloe: Yeah, I actually ran into him in town. He told me he was going to see a friend, but when he walked into the building I saw the sign for an oncologist.

Anna: So we wonder if he has cancer.

Marianne: But he said he was seeing a friend?

Chloe: No, but Mom he was really uncomfortable.

Marianne: Well, maybe for other reasons. I think he's in good shape. A little too much, even.

Anna: Well, maybe it's all just smoke and mirrors.

Marianne: No, I'll tell you why it's impossible for him to be sick.

Anna: Why?

Marianne: Because if he was sick the whole city would know, you, me, the neighbor's cat.

Anna: He likes to attract attention ok, but maybe not with such a serious disease.

Chloe: Professor Labose, do you know him?

Marianne: Well, yes, a little.

Chloe: Well, maybe you could ask him.

Marianne: No, but what about medical confidentiality?

Anna: But how do we know that then?

Marianne: Look, if he's sick and doesn't want to say so, that's his business.

Chloe: But Mom, you can't say something like that, we have to know if he's sick.

Marianne: But why?

Anna: But because you can't hide something that serious from your children.

Chloe: Well, obviously, and we want to be there to support him, to be with him. We need to know now if he's sick or not. Not once he's dead.

Marianne: Dealing with people who panic or feel sorry for you can be difficult too.

Anna: It's funny how you're reacting. You seem to know something.

Chloe: But of course she knows something. I'm sure Dad talked to her.

Marianne: Not at all! Well, girls, you're starting to bore me now. There's nothing wrong with him. I am a doctor and I know him well.

Chloe: Well, if you don't want to help us, that's okay. We'll ask him about it.

Marianne: Go ahead and do that[9].

The patient cannot and will not deal with her daughters' emotions such as fear, panic, pessimism and even less resentment. She explains to Renaud that she does not want them to worry and dramatize. Her choice to keep her cancer a secret from her daughters, which she claims, is challenged by her daughters when they learn the truth. She reminds them that she does not have to justify herself, because "in this story", she is the sick one and she says it if she wants, when she wants and to whom she wants…[10].

The illness splits a before and an after, thus constituting a biographical division, requiring the borrowing of another path whose intensity and experience force the individual to recompose their social identity. For the patient, it is a matter of "regaining a certain control over her biography and restoring social identity" (Francequin 2012, p. 167). This is exactly the process of reappropriation and recomposition that Marianne Delcourt goes through in the course of the narrative sequences devoted to her illness. The example of the ordeals experienced by the character in the series overlaps with the testimonies of the patients suffering from cancer. The analysis of these testimonies collected in the context of confessional programs from the 1980s to 2007 shows that what poses a problem are "the relationship between the couple (sexuality, dialogue, separation); the relationship with the family (telling the truth to the children, bearing the compassionate attitude of relatives); the self-image (hair and breast prostheses, body transformation). These three invariants of the testimonial make it possible to identify a sort of common background to the experience of the disease among sufferers" (Ceditec, INCa, 2010, p. 63).

---

9 Episode 386, aired on January 25, 2019, 10 mins 48 to 12 mins 38. At Marianne's house with her daughters Chloe and Anna.

10 Episode 401.

6.5. Conclusion

This type of narrative arc in the series raises socially sensitive issues related to intimacy and death. The characters of *Demain nous appartient* belong to a contemporary world in which they become flesh and the series proposes reflections on recurring themes, becoming a privileged place of social identification for the viewers:

> Like no other current media, the series have the capacity to develop complex worlds, which gives them the status of a contemporary "human comedy". Some of them allow us to explore, as a novel does, regions, cities, social environments as microcosms. The series thus form the volumes of a vast Human Comedy of the beginning of the 21st century, a multiform work, with multiple authors, a collective work. They are post-modern fables, exercises in morality (Damour 2015, pp. 81–92).

Although the television series *Demain nous appartient* does not explicitly pursue a learning goal, but rather an entertainment one, a lot of information on care is nevertheless staged. This is the case with French or American series featuring doctors or paramedics, which have achieved record ratings. Viewers seek to understand the care activity in dramatic situations. The scriptwriters are betting that the audience will adhere to the serial narrative insofar as it proposes vicarious models.

The recurring characters in these series have gained depth (Jost 2011). They present psychological characteristics (stereotypes and counter-stereotypes) that the viewer can feel close to (Crombet and Hélène 2017) or that give them food for thought. As Marc and Rose Nagels explain,

> From then on, empathy with the characters will arise, fostered by the anchoring of the action in reality and the tendency for social comparison. Viewers can recognize themselves in the characters, in their story, in their ability to withstand obstacles and in their ingenuity to solve problems. This is the case here with Marianne Delcourt,

her professional, family and emotional entourage. The analysis of the perceptions that viewers of series have refers to the processes of identification and projection to which the characters of the series can be subjected. The viewer's ability to identify with the character, to recognize them as a peer, is one of the conditions for successful vicarious learning (Bandura 2003, p. 43).

Vicarious learning is not based on a direct experience of the subject, but on that of their peers, in doing so, it facilitates the subject's entry into the activity through the analysis that the subject must make of the activity of their peers. In a social-cognitive approach to agentivity, i.e. the subject's ability to self-influence, influence others, and the environment, and social learning, video is an effective medium in a pedagogical strategy that consists of observing behaviors in order to deduce the underlying modes of action (Nagels and Nagels 2015).

Researchers have hypothesized that television series, in the form of videos that are easily accessible from home, help shape audience behavior. On a large scale, studies have been able to show the role played by television series (Singhal et al. 2004) in regulating birth control or preventing HIV.

The example of the relationship between the caregiver and the breast cancer patient in *Demain nous appartient* is a case in point. From the presentation of the disease, to the advice given for a quick and efficient management, the series seems to us to propose vicarious learning.

6.6. References

Aksakal, N. (2015). Theoretical view to the approach of the edutainment. *Procedia, Social and Behavioral Sciences*, 186, 1232–1239.

Bandura, A. (2003). *Auto-efficacité. Le sentiment d'efficacité personnelle*. De Boeck, Brussels.

Barthes, S. (2016). Panique à la télé : la résistance bactérienne vue par les séries télévisées. *Questions de communication*, 29, 111–134.

Belorgey, N., Pinsard, É., Rousseau, J. (2016). Naissance de l'aidant. Les pratiques des employeurs face à leurs salariés soutenant un proche. *Genèses*, 102(1), 67–88.

Bonneaudeau, S. (2011). Le médecin/malade, un patient comme les autres ? Thesis, Université Paris Diderot.

Boutet, M. (2019). Les séries, miroir des sociétés. *Éducation aux images et séries*, 54–70, Les éditions de l'Acap, Amiens.

Ceditec (2010). Le cancer dans les médias 1980–2007. Document, INCa.

Charon, R. (2015). *Médecine narrative, rendre hommage aux histoires de maladies*. Sipayat, Paris.

Chatel, T. (2010). Ethique du "prendre soin" : sollicitude, care, accompagnement. In *Traité de bioéthique*, Emmanuel, H. (ed.). Erès, Toulouse. DOI: halshs-00707121.

Corroy, L. (ed.) (2008). Un feuilleton hexagonal qui plaît : plus belle la vie. In *Les Jeunes et les médias, les raisons du succès*. Vuibert, Paris.

Crombet, H. (2021). Personnage de fiction. *Publictionnaire. Dictionnaire encyclopédique et critique des publics*. Published online 13 October 2017. Last modified 5 October 2021 [Online]. Available at: http://publictionnaire.huma-num.fr/notice/personnage-de-fiction.

Damour, F. (2015). Pourquoi regardons-nous les séries télévisées ? *Etudes*, 81–92.

Francequin, G. (ed.) (2012). *Cancer du sein : une féminité à reconstruire*. Erès, Toulouse.

Goupy, F. and Le Jeunne, C. (eds) (2016). *La médecine narrative. Une révolution pédagogique ?* Éditions Med Line, Paris.

Hochschild, R.A. (2017). *Le prix des sentiments, au coeur du travail émotionnel*. La Découverte, Paris.

Marche, H. (2020). A contra-intimité. Les mises en forme artistiques de la maladie grave. *Corps*, 18, 187–198.

Nagels, M. and Nagels, R. (2015). Comprendre et apprendre le soin à travers les séries télévisées, en France et au Liban. *Phronesis*, 3(4), 36–50.

Parat, H. (2017). Sein perdu, sein retrouvé. *Revue française de psychosomatique*, 51, 101–116.

Savignat, P. (2014). Les aidants : une catégorie incertaine entre domaine privé et espace public. *Empan*, 4(96), 151–157.

Singhal, A., Cody, M.J., Rogers, E.M., Sabido, S. (eds) (2004). *Entertainment-education and Social Change: History, Research and Practice.* Lawrence Erlbaum Associates Publishers, Hillsdale.

Soum-Pouyalet, F. (2006). Le risque émotionnel en cancérologie. Problématiques de la communication dans les rapports entre soignants et soignés. *Face à Face*, 8 [Online]. Available at: https://journals.openedition.org/faceaface/257.

Truc, H., Alderson, M., Thompson, M. (2009). Le travail émotionnel qui sous-tend les soins infirmiers : une analyse évolutionnaire de concept. *Recherche en soins infirmiers*, 2(97), 34–49.

WHO (2011). Patient Safety Curriculum Guide, Multi-professional Edition. WHO, Report.

7

Taming Cancer. Affected Bodies, Mirrored Emotions and Challenges for Patients and Their Loved Ones

Although the status of a carer is increasingly recognized in French legislation, the interventions of relatives throughout the patient's trajectory remain partially known and/or poorly understood by health professionals. Analysis of the material from the CORSAC study (*COoRdination des Soins Ambulatoires durant la phase thérapeutique initiale du Cancer*), including the role of relatives, reveals implicit and incomplete aspects of cancer care. The various individual challenges are not the same according to the knowledge of experience and social groups. The least well-to-do patients can rely more on their relatives to cope with everyday life and show strategic withdrawals that are similar to genuine empowerment.

7.1. Introduction – a limited recognition of the role of relatives?

One French person in 10 helps a loved one with cancer, this help being related to treatment compliance, accompaniment to medical appointments and chemotherapy sessions as well as to the daily life of the sick person (administrative tasks, help with housework, shopping and cooking, washing and dressing). In addition to psychological support and maintaining social ties, the majority of caregivers provide "financial assistance to their sick loved one, most often to compensate for the loss

Chapter written by Anne VEGA and Ibtissem BEN DRIDI.

of income" (*Report by the Observatoire sociétal des cancers*, 2016[1]). This assistance is often essential to their survival (Kroenke et al. 2006).

In connection with this, there has been a movement in France to recognize the status of a caregiver. The law on the adaptation of society to aging, which came into force in 2016, now even recognizes the role of caregivers as complementary to that of professionals. These developments are in line with those of "domestic *care*" (Damamme and Paperman 2009; Papadaniel et al. 2016) and the healthcare system. More and more people are going to HDJs (day hospitals), where we chose to recruit most of the respondents in the CORSAC collective survey (see Box 7.1). The growing increase in activity in oncology day hospitals has resulted in a decrease in contact time with caregivers. In other words, the home – where we also conducted interviews – has become a place of care in its own right: with a transfer of "part of the medical work to the patient himself" (Ménoret 2015) and/or to "family and professional caregivers at home" (Saillant and Boulianne 2003). Our survey confirms the extent to which care, its organization and its effects are most often endorsed by relatives. However, the persistent gaps between the "rhetoric of the patient at the center of discourse" and their actual involvement (Mougeot et al. 2018) seem to be even more marked with regard to the patient's relatives in the practices we observed.

We will first show why relatives are brought to play a representative role of (para)medical care. This first part, which will allow a temporal perspective of the social support and assistance received on a daily basis by the patients, will be followed by a brief presentation of why caregivers distance themselves or need to do so. We will then present our specific results. Patients encountering cancer for the first time have to tame it, hence the importance of support from their families and friends[2]. And patients from working-class to

---

1 See: https://www.ligue-cancer.net/vivre/article/37632_les-aidants-ces-combattants-tres-discrets.

2 "The role of the friendship network has become considerable, and in many cases it is taking the place of the family link" (Hubert, 2006: 229), especially when the patients surveyed are single. We might add that relatives are referred to as friends, and vice versa: best friends are referred to as "sisters" or "brothers"; health or social sector professionals can also be or become friends.

disadvantaged backgrounds – socially and/or economically – are confronted with an accumulation of difficulties, hence the need for extended interventions by relatives, including the solidarity of their kin[3], and/or their (former) colleagues, as well as "acquaintances" (sometimes including patient caregivers, and/or members of their community).

This chapter is based on a collective survey CORSAC ("*COoRdination des Soins Ambulatoires durant la phase thérapeutique initiale du Cancer*") carried out by observations and in-depth interviews either in the presence of relatives, or during which the question of relatives/caregivers was expressly addressed. The study began in 2011 in cancer centers (CLCCs) (Corsac 1) and was extended in 2015 to public hospitals (Corsac 2), which are the place of care for the majority of patients undergoing chemotherapy. A third fieldwork, still financed by the INCa (French Cancer Institute), is underway in the French overseas territories (Corsac 3): to date, more than 126 interviews have been conducted with patients and/or their families. In the cancer centers, recruitment included patients with the four most common cancers, before extending our protocol to all cancers, in connection with the issue of social inequalities in health. Indeed, the objective of this research is to give an account of the patients' view of their disease and their medical care, by also bringing out the voice of people in socioeconomic difficulties. In line with this comprehensive and global approach, interviews were also conducted with the caregivers of the patients interviewed.

Box 7.1. *Methodology*

7.2. The invisible work of family caregivers in the care trajectory of the patient

Following the example of the first two editions of the national VICAN survey (Le Corroller-Soriano et al. 2008; INCa 2014), relatives have forcefully imposed themselves onto us in the field, both as witnesses and actors in the management of the disease, and throughout

---

3 That is, "all the people with whom the individual is related (blood relatives, allies, in-laws through recomposition) [constituting a] network of sociability and mutual aid" (Déchaux 2009, p. 91).

the care pathway. In light of the literature, three aspects of their "work"[4] remain underestimated by the professionals taking care of them.

7.2.1. *Memorizing and/or translating and coordinating consultations*

Relatives appear at the time of diagnosis announcements, episodes that are prominent in people's testimonies: synonymous with rupture, collapse of reference points (a "sideration" effect also widely described in the literature), or an "endless circle" for people in recurrence having more difficulty "coping" with the side effects of chemotherapy and lacking "both information about their treatment and the lethal threat linked to the presence of metastases" (Camara 2017). The result of all this is an inability or difficulty in understanding and/or recording what the doctor says during the consultation, and a relay taken by the relative. The latter then takes on the role of memorizing the medical discourse, which they will generally keep throughout the illness, ensuring the continuity of the subject over time; all the more so as the patient is often confronted with memory loss and changing medical interlocutors in day hospitals (organization of care not very conducive to "personalized follow-up"). Moreover, during our interviews, patients frequently asked their partners or siblings for confirmation of certain medical identities, as well as treatment time frames. Relatives also participated in understanding and/or translating medical jargon, even if it meant looking for information on the Internet (a role often taken on by the children of the patients surveyed).

A final aspect of the work remains spontaneously and collectively assumed (Vega 2014): the coordination of care between the different medical consultations and/or the social sector. Relatives establish the link between the different hospital services, between the hospital and the city, between doctors and non-doctors and/or between official and "non-conventional" medicine. Indeed, care is still often segmented or fragmented, hence the need to help manage medical records, which the patients themselves must update and bring to the various doctors.

---

4 According to the Straussian approach, which makes it possible to problematize the disease around the "work" necessary for its management, whether this work is carried out by professionals, by the patient themselves or by their entourage.

7.2.2. *Accompanying: trying to reduce anxiety, restoring image and dignity*

Other consequences of the organization of care are that relatives often physically accompany the respondents during their examinations and/or treatments: sometimes out of principle and/or duty (see the next point), but above all because of difficulties in getting to the appointment times set for the treatments and unpredictable waits that are often considered "demoralizing" in day hospitals (Vega 2014). Indeed, waiting for chemotherapy alongside people in a very poor state of health and coming across children affected by cancer can have a lasting effect on both patients and those accompanying them: "the number of people who come to receive these products is unbelievable [...] there are mostly women [...] The worst thing is the children" (husband of a patient, cancer center).

However, caregivers do not always dare to tell their sick loved one about the mental burden and significant fatigue: like caregivers who "take it upon themselves", they have to control themselves, go back and/or repress their own emotions. A man accompanying his sick wife explains:

> I can't even tell you [...] I was, uh... a wreck! A wreck, that I was [...] But I was ashamed, I was ashamed [...] If I was tired, what was she feeling with her chemotherapy?

Indeed, during the period of the beginning of the treatments,

> the sometimes violent or trivializing vocabulary, the rapid sequence of examinations, the contradiction of the medical discourse and even the atmosphere of the care are described by the patient as particularly anxiety-provoking (Bounié 2018).

The support offered at this stage is biomedical ("it's protocol, protocol") and/or depersonalized ("we are numbers").

In any case, the uncertain character of the effects of the treatments and/or the etiologies is often the cause of anxiety that invades the treated persons when they return home because of important fluctuations of "morale", temporal disorientation, slowing down of thought, or other cognitive disorders that are not yet medically recognized; to which can be added the image of a diminished body and mind.

For the relatives, it is then a matter of temporizing, or even positivizing – borrowing para-medical strategies to maintain the patient's morale (Vega and Soum Pouyalet 2010) – even if the experience of deterioration is experienced simultaneously alongside the person being cared for: "my wife was Picasso"[5].

Most relatives tend to reassure, to reduce the image of the disease that takes over the body and/or to help with mourning. This is the case, for example, of a young childless patient who was having difficulty mourning the loss of her fertility, helped by her older sister[6]. In these situations, bodily touch can participate in the "little things that change everything" according to patients: to feel that a hand warms one's own at night, to have massages of the face or scalp, etc. The re-sexualization of the body is also often an important step, with the many rituals at the end of treatment that also involve accompanying people on trips, spa treatments, etc.

When the patient is no longer able to move around, the family member organizes visits to the patient: which people are authorized to enter the privacy of the room? To what extent does the patient accept the disclosure of their sick body to others? At the end of life at home, part of the role of the family member becomes clearer to the professionals who come to the bedside. Relatives – including the elderly – take on certain technical caregiving tasks, without having been prepared or trained for them. However, some people say that they take on these tasks better than any other caregivers because they try to respect the particularities of their loved one. For example, a sick woman, a former doctor, cannot stand having medication put directly into her mouth. Her former status as a doctor means that she needs to

5 Excerpts from the Corsac 1 material where caregivers were often the husbands of breast cancer patients.

6 Corsac 2 (pre-report online: https://annevega.files.wordpress.com/2021/03/pre-rapport-corsac-2.pdf).

control the medication she ingests. In all cases, remaining "dignified" in illness is one of the leitmotifs that comes up in most of the interviews, hence the need to guard against the pity of others.

7.2.3. (Re)building or unraveling relationships: limits to commitments

While there is also an abundance of literature on the reconfiguration of relationships between cancer patients and their loved ones, the parallel between the latter and the ways in which caregivers act also seems to be an instructive line of work. Indeed, caring means making a personal commitment, and the variety of positions (empathy/avoidance) is related to the representations and emotions that caregivers arouse in patients (Vega 2012b). Thus, cancer announcements go hand in hand with the resumption of contact by former friends, previous mates, relatives – opportunities for mutual rediscovery, "beautiful encounters" often unexpected by patients. Commitments are reaffirmed: "I tell him: 'I'm afraid you'll look elsewhere' – because it happened to me once; he told me: 'but you have nothing to fear: when I'm committed to someone I'm committed'."

On the other hand, the distancing, defection and/or abandonment by relatives seem to be linked to their own apprehension of death, or even to the idea that the illness/misfortune is contagious ("The family does not dare come, can you imagine?! Because they are afraid of disturbing, because they are afraid". Patient in metastatic relapse). This can happen even within a sibling group, where some members withdraw from accompanying the parent as soon as a relative takes care of them. But more often, avoidance occurs in a wider circle, involving distant family members, friends (renamed "false friends" by the patients) or neighbors. The reason given by these people is that they do not feel capable of handling the emotional burden of care and/or wish to keep a "good image" of the sick relative.

Sometimes relatives are therefore in a relationship of avoidance and refuse to see the diminished person. But mirror effects also operate on the side of the patient. The sick person may refuse help from family members (and family members may interpret this as a sign that the person being cared for does not trust them) because of the image that they do not want to inflict on family members, which offends their own modesty: "I'm sorry you see me like this", "And to think that everyone sees me in this decrepit state!". The need to take time off for themselves[7] – *especially* when they are free from the injunction to fight and stay strong – also explains the distance taken by patients. "I would have preferred to be alone at that time [...] My friend says: 'As long as you hold on, I'll hold on'. Maybe I don't want to hold on... Maybe I want to let go, maybe I don't want to be okay...". Finally, some patients prefer to share their experiences with other patients following misunderstandings, or by excluding their relatives out of kindness (so as not to "wear them out", "not to hurt those around me"), especially when they invest too much: "I would have asked for the moon, they would have gone to get it [...] and I don't like it". As with the announcements, the logic of preserving one's loved ones and preserving oneself is often intertwined. For example, one patient hid her cancer from her parents when she began treatment: they lived abroad and

> I was afraid for my mother's morale and mental health [...], I honestly didn't have the strength or the courage to deal with my parents' worries.

If, afterwards, a complex dynamic is put in place (each one trying to put on a good face, or even not to "*let* anything *show*"), the ideal for the patient is to be able to select relatives by selective affinities:

> When I'm in a slump, I have a sister [...] she lived through her husband's cancer and then [...] Since we're brother and sister, mentally, we're pretty much the same. Let's just say that she knows the words to help me find my courage; if I don't see her crack, it gives me strength. And she, if she doesn't see me break down, it gives her strength too because she also had cancer.

---

7 Which can also be done through diaries (to assimilate, "*accept the hard blow*", find oneself, "*draw strength*" from oneself).

Among women, we often observe the careful constitution of networks of female allies, including family friends (Vega 2012a). This is because it is a question of not asking too much of the men in the family, including spouses who are likely to "fall apart", brothers and fathers who are less socialized to care ("I don't want moral support, that's all. If I really need someone, it's really a help – we'll say practical").

7.3. The centrality and vitality of caregivers

In the same way that there are major differences between caregivers who have or have not encountered cancer, there are also major differences between patients with no experience of cancer, including among their relatives ("first-time cancer patients"), and those who had already undergone serious episodes of health disruption (hospitalization before the cancer) and/or had accumulated a certain amount of expertise about their disease during their treatment. These patients are more assertive with both doctors and their relatives. As for patients belonging to well-to-do to very well-to-do social backgrounds in the study, they traditionally use inter-knowledge networks of people with the same level of education as oncologists to improve their care: to be treated more quickly, to be listened to more, to promote negotiation and coordination of their care (Hardy 2013; Camara 2017; Barthe and Defossez 2021)[8]. In other cases, faced with the accumulation of difficulties to manage in addition to the disease, family and extended supports take on other dimensions.

7.3.1. *To have ties and networks of medical inter-knowledge*

For "first-time cancer patients", "you have to learn how to manage". Managing the disease involves learning the medical vocabulary, the organization of care and taming the disease. Cancer is often perceived as an invisible, chaotic and truly threatening entity when the patient is socially isolated, as was shown in the *Nurses'*

8 And vice versa: the most "vulnerable" people are the first victims of coordination failures, according to the director of quality at Gustave-Roussy (*8èmes rencontres de la cancérologie française*, December 15–16, 2015, Paris).

Health Study (cited in C.H. Kroenke et al. 2006). Conversely, primary caregivers who have ties know that they are vital: "At least I am well surrounded"; "I get along very well with my children, thank God they are here"; "Without my two daughters, I would not be here for a long time". The relationship that the primary caregiver has with the sick family member often becomes a very intimate one. Moreover, in interviews conducted in pairs, they generally express themselves in the plural: "We have tamed the disease", "we have managed to overcome the disease".

Being "in the game" oneself, having a close friend who belongs to the medical profession can also bring clear improvements in care (Jourdain and Morel 2016). However, the lower the socioeconomic level, the less networks and knowledge people have of the world of health – medical and specialized a fortiori: the least well-to-do respondents are less able to be heard or be informed, to negotiate or reframe medical consultations (Fainzang 2006; Vega 2012b; Gelly and Pitti 2016). In other words, these respondents have submissive relationships with the healthcare system and biomedicine (Byron Good 1994). They have at the same time more respect, trust and fear towards doctors, with whom they can generally negotiate less: because of a cultural distance to the medical world, as well as because of the lack of consistent social networks. In fact, only a minority of patients' relatives dared to intervene in healthcare relationships in the last two parts of the CORSAC study. On the other hand, they faced other barriers, both epidemiological and social.

7.3.2. *Having administrative and financial assistance*

Cancer remains a "socially selective scourge", triggered in 2/3 of cases by environmental factors external to the physiology of each person (Derbez and Rollin 2016), contributing to the earlier onset of cancers in the least favored social groups[9]. The latter are treated to a greater extent in public establishments, which combine the care of the incurable and most serious cancers with that of the elderly. In fact, recruitment is often carried out in the vicinity of or in connection with

---

9 See: http://invs.santepubliquefrance.fr/beh/2017/4/pdf/2017_4_1.pdf.

"pockets of working-class and precarious environments" – including people of foreign origin and/or "undocumented" – which are also known to reduce cancer survival rates. In other words, people who are generally in poorer health before cancer often arrive with worse cancers, and experience greater fatigue and pain that is not always expressed.

The main difficulties encountered by these respondents focus first and foremost on the administrative procedures that they must often carry out during their treatment, especially since they are not always helped by social workers (insufficient in number, "not very much in the loop", and/or reluctant to take care of "foreigners"). However, the financial question – including the advance payment of expenses and out-of-pocket expenses – is central in the testimonies of patients and their relatives. For example, the costs of television, hospital parking spaces and/or Internet connection weighed more heavily for some families, to which was added the cost of wigs and specialized clothing for women in metropolitan France. These difficulties sometimes weigh as much or even more than the location of the cancer, the treatments received or the perceived after-effects (Le Corroller-Soriano et al. op. cit.), and family relatives are more involved in medical care: via financial aid and accommodation, in the management of administrative files – including by entering into conflict with hospital social workers. As in other chronic pathologies, they take on the role of representing the patient and providing moral support, since these steps are often exhausting (Braud 2017). For example, a young Algerian patient living with her sister was in debt to the tune of 2,000 euros (following the purchase of a box costing more than 1,000 euros), as her Pass card only covered hospital care. She also did not receive any help during the first four months of her treatment for her public transport to the hospital, and it was her sister who contacted the social services to reaffirm and finally obtain her rights.

7.3.3. *Behind the duty to support: helping keep morale up, social utility and trying to survive*

Close and extended families have particularly helped patients of foreign origin financially to cover the costs of care and/or multiplied the steps taken before their relative could benefit from 100% coverage, residence permits or "green cards", AME[10] and/or mutual insurance. However, whatever the cultural origins of the respondents, people treated in the public sector often have to deal with physical, psychological and social after-effects. In the face of adversity, it is above all a question of keeping their spirits up at all costs, which is at the heart of the strategies of the family members surveyed, including religious support ("My family also prays for me"). This explains the refusal to use psychologists because they are considered "useless", as well as "demoralizing". Moreover, the support of relatives helps to remove or attenuate the discrepancies between the "good" practices promoted by the ARS[11], and living conditions. For how can we adapt to the injunctions to "eat well" or healthily (a marker of social inequalities[12]), to do sports, to participate in supportive care, in organized events and now in "resilience coaching"? Most patients cannot access these practices because they are too costly and/or unsuitable for their deteriorating health. Relatives prepare "good meals" that are more appreciated by their patients than diets recommended by dietitians and/or use their networks to provide access to complementary or alternative therapies that are also more accessible and affordable[13].

Other recourse to and refusal of help outside the immediate family, resulting in an under-consumption of institutional services and outside help at home, cannot be explained solely by habits of endurance (more marked appreciation of "resisting evil"[14]). For example, one patient

---

10 The AME (*Aide Médicale de l'Etat*) is a system allowing foreigners in an irregular situation to have access to healthcare.

11 The Regional Health Agencies (ARS) are public establishments of an administrative nature, under direct ministerial supervision but with a degree of autonomy.

12 Whether these are understood in terms of monetary criteria (income, standard of living) or socio-professional criteria (diploma, profession): https://www.foodplanet.fr/app/download/5790614657/esco-inra-comportements-synthese.pdf.

13 See: http://journals.openedition.org/anthropologiesante/606.

14 "Everybody tells me that, actually: 'You're strong, you've got the drive, you've got the, you've got the... the will, you've got'... Uh.... But actually, I'm petrified uh... inside. But uh... I try not to show it to others".

explained that she did not ask for anything from outside her immediate family:

> We can't count, no, no, no [...] I don't want to! It's [that] my family, it's me and my children. In all my life, I've never asked for social services, so asking for help, I don't like that.

And their position is reinforced by experiences of administrative procedures that are too long and uncertain – more recently, the disability allowance at their expense, despite contacts with a hospital social worker.

> I think it's worth pfff! No – still breaking down doors, thinking about it, no no: I wanted to deal with it, to accept it – And it was likely to? – To be traumatic for me. All the steps, without knowing [if] it will work, not work. No, I want my health back.

This limited trust outside the family circle (Lacourse 2018) is therefore also to be understood as forms of social autonomy in the sense of François Dubet (1994, p. 17[15]). Not only does social assistance – like information in care – remain essentially based on the formulation of a request, but social assistance schemes expose people to new ordeals, while they do not want to wear out their "strengths" and seek to "keep face". More precisely, it is about not being seen as incompetent, as diminished or useless. Also, all genders and ages combined, the most important thing for the relatives of these respondents is also to help them to remain active and independent (to continue their occupations, to keep busy, to keep their home "clean"), even if this requires not intervening too much with the patient. This helps them to maintain a good image and even to give meaning to their lives – sources of mutual pride.

---

15 It is about the critical distance that the actors keep in front of the system and the reflexivity that they exercise, often "following feelings of suffering and alienation experienced when they do not manage to find meaning and to keep control of their actions in front of the variety of logics they are confronted with".

Whether willingly or not, empowerment is therefore achieved more between oneself and at home and/or in a home. And the notion of having to support our loved ones on a daily basis, which is more common among working-class families, appears to be an obvious obligation: "If you are ill, they are always with you and give you all the care and love you need". As for socially isolated patients, some benefit from broader support: friendships, between neighbors in the neighbourhood and/or with former work colleagues. However, they include people who are geographically isolated from their families due to health migration. Connected exchanges and "*home cooking*" sometimes prove insufficient, hence the importance of being able to bring one's family to stay on and

> "to have the courage to continue the treatments"; "without her, I couldn't do it, but I miss my family [crying]"; "I would at least like to see my mother again, besides she is sick"; "I haven't seen my children, they are small, for 1 year and I was told that their father doesn't take care of them anymore…" (Comorian patient treated in Mayotte).

In other words, defections such as the impossibility of traveling can also be the source of great moral suffering. Migrants from all social backgrounds are in fact in the hope of survival – although sometimes in the palliative stages of cancer. And it is these same logics that have motivated health migrations, the costs of which are traditionally assumed collectively to allow sick people to come to the Mayotte hospital center from the Comoros, for example – because they are very poor and there is no cancer treatment there. After arriving in *kwassa* (fishermen's boats), only some of these patients can benefit from medical evacuations to Reunion. In all these situations, the study shows at this stage the importance of associative relays and informal support from other Comorian patients as well as from health and/or social sector professionals.

7.4. Conclusion – helping to maintain dignity and morale: another form of empowerment to be recognized

If "the relatives are to be defined on a case-by-case basis, for each patient" (Hubert 2006, p. 229), in our interviews carried out in pairs with patients and relatives, the latter reiterate, translate, complete, nuance and/or re-establish the patient's words by helping them to remember and to coordinate their care. On this point, our survey confirms that the famous "bio-psycho-social" model (Rossi 2009) still appears to be a succession of juxtaposed actions by medical, paramedical and family workers, who remain "satelliteized", just like the social workers (Sainsaulieu and Vega 2014). Moreover, in France, the development of empowerment depends on the power to mobilize a family circle that "carries weight": explanations and negotiations become effective when people from a well-to-do social background are involved alongside the patient, a fortiori when there is "class complicity" with the medical community (Hardy, op. cit.). In the absence of these networks, sick people from "working-class" backgrounds and those with fewer resources are traditionally supported more by their family circle (Bataille 2003): both to "keep their spirits up" and remain dignified, and to cope with financial insecurity and administrative difficulties. Because of their deteriorating health and their distance from the world of healthcare, they rely more on doctors. But behind the apparent submission to medical authority and/or refusal of institutional help, the respondents show strategic withdrawal from relatives who care about them and seek appropriate solutions, including in relation to health injunctions that are impossible to achieve – because they take as a reference the behaviors of the most privileged social groups. For all these reasons, the family and close circle of friends, everyday people and/or members of community networks become essential to maintain the patient's social position and autonomy; indeed, they are the only possibilities for listening and supporting patients.

On all these points, our results to date are in line with those of sociologist Rosane Braud with diabetes patients in public hospitals. They describe caregivers:

> globally as the main source of support for their life with the disease. They are mobilized for a whole range of aspects of

life: management of administrative files and the search for
financial solutions where necessary, management of
therapy and diet, sharing of everyday tips for solving
a given problem related to therapy, development of
self-esteem, reinforcement of their enrolment in sociability
networks, listening when morale is low, etc. (Braud 2017,
p. 442).

At a time when, following the pandemic, WHO-Europe is
highlighting a growing number of "vulnerable" people, the notion of
caregiver should therefore be taken in a broad sense, to include all
those supporting and/or surrounding the patient, whose actions are
most often similar to care. However, the promotion of empowerment
operates at the expense of social and structural logics in health
(Bergeron and Castel 2014). Also, in practice, we observe in our care
institutions difficulties in the face of differences in support (Grangiens
2019), coupled with a hierarchization of patients as well as relatives:
according to their social status, their profession and/or their supposed
cultural origins. We will have to take a closer look at the limits placed
on the presence of carers by health and/or social sector professionals,
but referring a priori to negative categorization processes based on
their supposed lesser skills or incapacities.

7.5. References

Barthe, J.-F. and Defossez, A. (2021). Les inégalités d'accès aux ressources
par les réseaux personnels chez les patients atteints de cancer. *Revue
française des affaires sociales*, 4, 207–225.

Bataille, P. (2003). *Un cancer et la vie. Les malades face à la maladie.*
Balland, Paris.

Bergeron, H. and Castel, P. (2014). *Sociologie politique de la santé.* PUF,
Paris.

Bounié, A.-S. (2018). Les usages de l'hypnose des patients dans l'épreuve du
cancer. Master's 2, Université de Versailles Saint-Quentin-en-Yvelines.

Braud, R. (2017). Construction d'une catégorie de "migrants" dans les
actions de lutte contre les inégalités face au diabète en France. PhD
Thesis, Université Sorbonne Paris Cité.

Byron Good, J. (1994). *Medicine, Rationality, and Experience: An Anthropological Perspective*. Cambridge University Press, New York.

Camara, H. (2017). Perceptions des patientes en rechute métastatique de l'accompagnement soignant. Master's 2, Université de Versailles Saint-Quentin-en-Yvelines.

Damamme, A. and Paperman, P. (2009). Care domestique : des histoires sans début, sans milieu et sans fin. *Multitudes*, 37–38, 98–105.

Déchaux, J.-H. (2009). *Sociologie de la famille*. La Découverte, Paris.

Derbez, B. and Rollin, Z. (2016). *Sociologie du cancer*. La Découverte, Paris.

Dubet, F. (1994). *Sociologie de l'expérience*. Le Seuil, Paris.

Fainzang, S. (2006). *La relation médecins-malades : information et mensonge*. PUF, Paris.

Gelly, M. and Pitti, L. (2016). Une médecine de classe ? Inégalités sociales, système de santé et pratiques de soins. *Agone*, 58, 7–18.

Grangiens, M. (2019). Les soignants hospitaliers face aux familles roms. Master's 1, Université Dauphine.

Hardy, A.-C. (2013). Variations sociologiques sur le thème de la médecine. HDR, Université de Nantes.

Hubert, A. (2006). Les proches : le point de vue de l'anthropologue. *Revue francophone de psycho-oncologie*, 5–4.

INCa (2014). La vie deux ans après un diagnostic de cancer – De l'annonce à l'après cancer. Report, INCa, Collection Études et Enquêtes.

Jourdain, M. and Morel, S. (2016). S'automédiquer sous chimiothérapie ? *Colloque international AUTOMED*, L'automédication en question. Un bricolage social et territorialement situé, Nantes.

Kroenke, C.H., Kubzansky, L.D., Schernhammer, E.S., Holmes, M.D., Kawachi, I. (2006). Social networks, social support and survival after breast cancer diagnosis. *Journal of Clinical Oncology*, 24(7), 1105–1111.

Lacourse, M.-T. (2018). *Sociologie de la santé*. Chenelière Education, Quebec.

Le Corroller-Soriano, A.-G., Malavolti, L., Mermilliod, C. (eds) (2008). *La vie deux ans après un diagnostic de cancer, une enquête en 2004 sur les conditions de vie des malades*. La Documentation française, Paris.

Ménoret, M. (2015). La prescription d'autonomie en médecine. *Anthropologie & Santé*, 10. doi:10.4000/anthropologiesante.1665.

Mougeot, F., Robelet, M., Rambaud, C., Occelli, P., Buchet-Poyau, K., Touzet, S., Michel, P. (2018). L'émergence du patient-acteur dans la sécurité des soins en France. *Santé Publique*, 30(1), 73–81.

Papadaniel, Y., Berthod, M.-A., Brzak, N. (2016). Ni soignant ni patient : clarifier le rôle des proches dans la relation thérapeutique. *Revue médicale suisse*, 12, 2034–2036.

Rossi, I. (2009). L'accompagnement en médecine. Anthropologie d'une nécessité paradoxale. *Pensée plurielle*, 22(3), 111–122.

Saillant, F. and Boulianne, M. (2003). *Transformations sociales, genre et santé*. PU de Laval, Quebec/Paris.

Sainsaulieu, I. and Vega, A. (2014). Introduction à la revue. *Les Sciences de l'éducation. Pour l'ère nouvelle*, 47(3), 13–40.

Vega, A. (2012a). La mort, l'oubli et les plaisirs. *Anthropologie et santé*, 4. doi:10.4000/anthropologiesante.861.

Vega, A. (2012b). Positivisme et dépendance : les usages socioculturels du médicament chez les médecins généralistes français. *Sciences sociales et santé*, 30(3), 71–102.

Vega, A. (2014). Le point de vue de patientes sur la prise en charge en secteur ambulatoire. *Les Sciences de l'éducation*, 47(3), 13–40.

Vega, A. and Soum-Pouyalet, F. (2010). Entre rationalité scientifique et croyances individuelles. *Anthropologie & sociétés*, 34(3), 230–248.

8

About Long Illnesses. Family Caregivers: Actors and Producers of Care and Health. The Case of Algeria

Care activities for patients with chronic and long-term illnesses are essentially provided by relatives. The family is seen as a space where health is treated daily. When a close relative is ill, a family member will very often mobilize and take care of them for free. Thus, our questioning focuses on the various socio-health acts that the patient's relative deploys daily. Relying on the notion of medical work (Strauss 1992) to show that the sick relative or "helper" is led to become an actor and producer of care and health (Cresson and Metboul 2010). We have favored the qualitative approach centered on 28 semi-structured interviews (26 women, two men and four focus groups) socially diversified with relatives and patients in the city of Oran. The analysis of our material shows that the close relative who is the patient intervenes in the production of care and health. All of the latter's work is accomplished by a woman (daughter, sister) reflecting an unequal sexual division of labor. Taking care of the patient is considered a duty and the consequences also weigh heavily on the well-being of the patient's relative.

8.1. Introduction

This chapter attempts to highlight the different socio-sanitary tasks presented to close relatives of those suffering from chronic and long-term illnesses. Caring for the sick is understood as a set of unrecognized and gratuitous tasks rooted in the social–gender relations throughout society. It is inconspicuous and taken for granted

Chapter written by Aicha BENABED.

as natural. It is ensured mainly within the family. A member of the family is often designated by expressions such as "sick nurse", "patient's relative" or "family carer" to distinguish them from the nursing staff who provide care within the framework of a standardized paramedical profession based on knowledge and rules.

Let us also note that the sociologist Alain Blanc (2010, p. 1) defines "family carers" as people from the family or being close to them having any lasting activity concerning a person being cared for characterized by a notable and lasting reduction in their capacities and skills. In fact, in this study, by the caregiver we mean all the people who voluntarily devote themselves to a loved one suffering from a chronic illness and often losing their autonomy. We use the terms "caregiver" and "patient's relative" as two identical terms. Because often the patient refers to the various social resources available in their close entourage to help them deal with complex and restrictive situations. It is therefore the family, as the "therapy organizing group" in the sense given by Janzen (1995, p. 16), which appears as a relational resource of prime importance for the patient. It is through this group that important decisions in terms of health are taken into account, especially for a patient who is unable to make their own decisions.

Thus, we start from an idea that defines chronic illness as a social event that affects the patient's social life in its entirety (Baszanger 1986). Chronic sickness is far from being a purely organic disorder. It is part of an open scheme that puts the patient in situations marked by uncertainty and rambling, and in a social dynamic characterized by a reorganization and a relational readjustment that is significant in the patient's social life. It is characterized by its disorganizing impact that affects all spheres of the patient's social life.

Patients' relatives are social actors who are capable of applying their experiential knowledge in the face of the illness of a close relative suffering from a chronic and/or long-term illness. Their knowledge can shed light on the use of medical knowledge, which can only be achieved by taking into account the practices of these sick relatives.

For this purpose, we rely on the qualitative approach based on 28 semi-structured and in-depth interviews (26 women, 2 men) and four socially diverse focus groups of patients' relatives who take care of their ill close relatives in Oran. The examples cited for this work relate much more to close relatives with their patients suffering from cancer, diabetes and Alzheimer's disease.

This methodological approach is relevant for accessing what the actors say and do, to understand how they construct their social reality. It updates the socially constructed discourses of particular versions of a lived reality. According to Beaud and Weber (2003), the purpose of this methodology is therefore the search for meaning, interpretations of reality constructed by individuals or the understanding of logical action. These caregivers are often women (daughter, spouse, sister, mother, daughter-in-law) aged between 28 and 47 years old.

Our research perspective focuses on the work of Cresson (1993) and Mebtoul (2005), which shows that both the patient's relative and the patient are decisive actors in the daily care activity, strongly refuting the "naturalization" of this health work that belongs to the social construct operated for the benefit of the patients by the health institution and society but without being socially recognized by health officials. This approach makes it possible to place the patient and the family at the center of the trajectory of the chronic disease as actors in the medical work necessary to maintain the patient's life.

The interest of this work deals with home care activities that are closer to the field. The elements that emerge from this study are structured as follows. First, we will try to give a brief overview of family help in the Algerian context. Second, we will discuss lay care as an alternative to medical work. We will show a set of profane socio-sanitary tasks produced by the patient's relative. Third, the motivation for which taking care of the patient becomes an obligation assimilated to duty and debt. Finally, we conclude by addressing the impact of care activities on the health of patients' relatives, which is described as a source of discomfort and fragility. The consequences weigh heavily on the well-being of the carer.

8.2. Family help in the Algerian context

> Health policies recognize the role of relatives and the
> burden of support that they endure, with which the
> relative is associated with actions relating to the patient
> and benefits from special attention, by taking their needs
> into account, of his or her suffering and the burden he or
> she bears in supporting the patient sick with chronic
> illness (cancer) (Kane et al. 2018, p. 39).

But this is not the case for Algeria, because family help as
professionalization has not yet seen the light of day. For many families,
it is difficult to turn a private issue into a social issue. This affects the
intimacy and confidentiality of their private life. We can mention the
mutual aid activities carried out by the volunteers of the associations
both in the hospital and at home. The study by Benkada and Metboul
(2018) shows that the non-profit work of volunteers makes it possible to
continue to take care of the patient, demonstrating various skills, each
according to their position. Their secular care work close to that of the
family remains invisible and unrecognized.

Indeed, the family has long been considered marginal with regard
to "triumphant medicine", the sole bearer of the power to treat
(Cresson and Mebtoul 2006). The relatives who accompany the
patient are often considered to be disruptors of the activities of health
professionals and carriers of diseases (nosocomial infections). The
Circular of the Ministry of Health No. 013 of January 27, 2007 was
issued to prohibit the presence of family members with patients. This
situation of non-compliance with family visiting hours from 1 p.m. to
3 p.m. is likely to disrupt care activities; it also constitutes a cause of
embarrassment and discomfort or even a risk of contamination for
hospital patients. Nevertheless, at different times in the patient's
trajectory, relatives are called upon to make up for certain
shortcomings of the hospital, for example, the purchase of some drugs
necessary for treatment, the provision of small items of medical
equipment (specific syringes, compresses, etc.) or the organization of
a blood drive to ensure the smooth running of the management of the
disease or to wash the patient. "Caregivers" mobilize to take care of
the patient and get involved in daily activities on a regular and

permanent basis. They take care of all domestic activities, treatment management, financial management, social life support, administrative procedures, psychological support, etc., to provide them with comfort and soothe their suffering.

Despite social changes, especially the generalization of nuclear families, which has promoted the isolation of their elderly patients suffering from long illnesses by placing them in institutions for the elderly, some caregivers have maintained their presence at home and take care of them. Our interlocutors refuse to consider the placement of their elderly parents and/or those suffering from chronic diseases or loss of autonomy in these institutions. This represents the worst curse for them, even though they are aware that the situation deserves more thought and attention. They highlight all the difficulties related to space, cramped buildings, lack of elevators, etc. They find it difficult to meet the expenses of their trip for consultations, although care is free for all chronic illnesses.

In addition, health officials are announcing the creation of geriatric hospitals but are reluctant to put them into practice for fear that families will neglect their sick relatives. They are announcing the lack of home help services to relieve families while providing care adapted to the needs of elderly patients with a loss of autonomy and disabilities. The withdrawal of the state in the field of care is contributing to the rediscovery of these caregivers as producers of health and care for the benefit of patients suffering from chronic diseases. Public authorities favor hospitalization at home for certain chronic patients to allow the free mobilization of family resources by granting some of their members the status of "caregiver" to reduce hospital expenditure and the burden of patients in the structures. This is what Bachimot (1998) showed when he said: "home hospital care contributes to home medicalization". These caregivers still retain an idealized perception of the traditional family perceived as having "more intergenerational solidarity". Despite the social changes experienced by the Algerian family, the way of conceiving family ties has not changed. The family remains a stable foundation. It is a strong claim and an ideal that is always desired.

8.3. Family help and secular care: an alternative to medical work

The work of the carer with their sick relative takes place discreetly and in the background of socially valued medical work. Numerous works in the sociology of health have made it possible to show the importance of the participation of sick relatives in carrying out care work accomplished throughout the trajectory of the disease and even well before a diagnosis is made. The activity of care is inseparable during the trajectory of the chronic patient who is the very pivot of its progress (Waisman 1995). Anselm Strauss (1992) focused most of his research on the ethnographic analysis of the concept of "medical work", in particular the different types of work involved in the trajectory of chronic illness. According to him, medical work includes not only the medical and paramedical activities necessary for the control and management of chronic diseases, but also all the other activities of care and support for the patient in the medical and family space.

As an example, we can mention the example of 28-year-old Malika who dedicated her life to helping her 7-year-old brother with cancer and her 45-year-old father with diabetes (and an amputated foot). This woman's experience shows that the patient's relative participates in the care of the patient suffering from a chronic illness, especially cancer, as soon as the first symptoms appear.

In the example of cancer, the multiple therapeutic itineraries strongly indicate that this woman participates in the production of health through the permanent quest for diagnosis and cure of her brother. This young girl is the first interlocutor in the observation of pain. She assesses the intensity of the pain. This shows that the process followed to find and diagnose the illness of this adolescent involves several doctors and specialists. She does a job of interpreting the symptoms according to their degree of severity by developing a hierarchy of serious or mild signs: for example, with the appearance of spots on the body, fever, headache and vomiting, this leads the young woman to identify the child's condition as pathological. Thus, the sudden onset of a worrying sign leads her to relaunch a search for care. Health activity is based on a cognitive posture that seems natural to them but is essential to inform health personnel. Observing, listening and memorizing the patient's complaints, are all resources mobilized by this woman during the monitoring work in the domestic space and even in the hospital. This woman performs medical work that "requires learning sophisticated techniques leading to know-how and knowledge about the disease, due to the accumulation of medical and practical knowledge" (Waissman 1995, p. 83). She becomes the main caregiver first within the family space and then in the hospital structure, where she continues to perform technical gestures such as cleaning the oral cavity with chemotherapy serums, changing dressings, etc.

Here are some illustrated excerpts:

> I had to give up my studies to take care of my family. I observed that he complained of tingling in his feet. He was having difficulty urinating … he has trouble walking, and he woke up in the morning with headaches and vomiting. I prepare tranquillizers and herbal teas for him. The doctor told me it was a growth problem, I wasn't convinced, so I took him to a second specialist, who gave the same answer. He had the same signs as our neighbor's son when I read on the internet that it could be cancer … but I didn't want to admit that, I accompanied him to a third specialist, he told me that it was articular rheumatism. But one evening, he had severe pain and unbearable cramps despite all the tranquillizers he had taken, he stayed awake, he did not sleep. When I saw him like that, I called the firefighters. They immediately took him to the emergency room. When they arrived at the emergency room, they gave him painkillers. They sent me to the hospital. In the morning at the hospital, my brother could no longer walk. He had paraplegia. He had a CT scan at a private hospital. The result revealed a malignant tumor, and the diagnosis of the tumor: was a stage 3 neuroblastoma. He was operated on in the same week in the neurosurgery department. Now we are in Misserghine at the anti-cancer center for cures.

At the same time, the help provided by this young woman is not limited to the usual household tasks. She helps her father daily and regularly to get up, dress, wash, eat, monitors him, observes, etc. She has to face the new situation caused by the onset of her father's illness. The help given to her diabetic father is characterized by various acts of care and very technical gestures, namely: measuring blood sugar, "calculating" the types and doses of insulin to be injected, and recognizing and acting in the face of hypoglycemia or hyperglycemia, preparing and controlling his diet, and preventing and monitoring his condition in case of complications.

Here is an example of such an illustration:

> [...] I have to do everything, at home and outside ... taking care of my brother and also my sister who is preparing her BEF... she wants to be a doctor, and so, the day I fall ill, she'll be the one who will take care of us... I have to take care of my father, monitor his diabetes, take care of his diet, and accompany him to the doctor. She says: "The blood pressure goes up to 20 and sometimes it goes down"... I give him his injection, it was a neighbour, a nurse who died more than twenty years ago, she was the one who showed me how to do it (Malika, 30 years old, bac +2 in law).

Care activities are socially constructed and reveal a distribution of gendered activities because it is essentially carried out by women. They deploy invisible skills that are rarely considered as a fair measure by other family members or health professionals. The active involvement of the patient's relative in taking care of their close relative makes it possible to identify their role as actors of care, holders of experiential knowledge and producers of diversified profane socio-sanitary practices.

They carry out support work in the hospital space. For example, 43-year-old Naima comes with her 67-year-old mother, who has pancreatic cancer, to get a CT scan at a private clinic on the second floor. The mother walks with difficulty leaning on her granddaughter. She moans in pain. Arriving on the first floor, Naima carries her mother in her arms as if she were carrying a 10-year-old child. She leads her to the waiting room. She helps her sit on the chair.

Here is an excerpt from the speech exchanged between the daughter and her mother:

> **Mother**: … I have six children, I always rely on my children to help me manage the various problems of my illness, but there is only one, it is Naima, who is regularly available … because her two brothers work, her two sisters are married in Tlemcen and the last is a university student, … her sisters only rarely come to see me but the most important thing for me is that I find them by my side … But Naima is present all the time. Naima without her, I'm dead … I don't exist … everything stops … She watches over me, gives me medicine, food, bathes me, she accompanies me to the doctors, to the hospital, she helps me to overcome the pain, she is like my psychologist, very close to me, she supports me when I get angry, she listens to me, she hugs me … her presence gives meaning to my life, thank God!

> **Naima**: Oh! Mama, come on! What I do with you is natural!

> **Mother**: No, my daughter! Everything has a price… You will be rewarded one day. If it's not in this world, you'll have it in heaven!

The various tasks performed at home seem to be natural, routine, ordinary and mundane. They are provided by a family member in their various social and sanitary spaces. This member becomes the primary helper at the heart of care work. Its active investment constitutes a psychological, health and social resource of primary importance for the patient. Care work is mainly assigned to women. In general, the man limits himself to financial support. The patient will be cared for by either the spouse, the mother, the sister, the daughter or even the daughter-in-law (Mebtoul 2010). Men too can perform all profane gestures and care. There is nothing "natural" that prevents them from doing so. But as soon as they have a woman in their homes (the daughter or the sister), she is therefore mainly considered to be available. The management of the disease by close relatives is mainly ensured by women, thus showing a gendered distribution of acts of care.

In addition, for patients who are both elderly and suffering from Alzheimer's disease, the carer is obliged not to separate from this relative who has become dangerous to themselves and others.

The patient with Alzheimer's disease is subject to behavioral problems. Risk in the field of mental health is generally related to the concepts of danger and threat or loss. Therefore, becoming a caregiver means adopting a new role, that of "being the parent to one's own parent". These caregivers are mostly women. Many are single, available every day and have unique skills in caring for their patients with Alzheimer's disease. These women play a fundamental role in taking care of their loved one who is weakened by age and illness or disability.

The presence of the caregiver provides a form of protection and security for the patient, both physically and psychologically. Something rarely mentioned with regard to care work is that of the risk of desocialization. Indeed, the image of dementia in society can cause a gradual cutting off of external relationships to close in the family, associated with a form of guilt or shame. However, some relatives will act differently.

Nadia, 45 years old, is single. She gave up her marriage plans to take care of her sick 70-year-old father, and tells us:

> I like that my father goes out to see people, his friends, even being sick, he needs contact, to be sociable, but it's difficult and it's risky, so you have to reverse things … it's my brother who takes care of the invitations…More or less these people know his disease, they try to reactivate and reflect his memory…by telling old anecdotes, good memories, moments of laughter, around a coffee, eating together, watching a football match…

People with family, friends, a close neighborhood or even professional relationships (ex-colleagues) constitute a relational capital thanks to which they are invited to share moments of conviviality with the patient in their home. These people are the same age as the patient and sometimes younger than them.

> I feel he is still insecure. I must be present at all times, and not lose sight of him. It's been almost six months since he opened the door and left the house… an hour later, we found out that he had had a car accident… (crying). He had a slight femur fracture… he was bedridden for a few months… bedsores appeared but not too serious, I was afraid of the risk of bedsores, because they can cause more serious and even fatal problems…I make honey-based dressings to treat bedsores, wash the wound with serum and cover it with honey and hold the dressing with a bandage before his doctor gives him morphine. I make him move his body, I change his position to relieve the pressure on the bedsores… I have to watch him because he gets nervous and restless…

The patient's relative provides prevention strategies that promote the patient's well-being. They mobilize all the know-how that they have learned over the course of their experience in the face of chronic illness. They can acquire real expertise and sometimes technical knowledge. For example, faced with the harmful effects of bedsores, the patient adopts a number of practices to strengthen weak muscles and replace inactive muscles by moving the body carefully and preventing the occurrence of bedsores, in particular by avoiding prolonged pressure on sensitive areas.

It seems that family help translates into so-called natural solidarity between family members. Those who do not live with their relatives can take over when the main person who takes care of their close relative is sick. It is generally the sister or the daughter who replaces them. Even if they are geographically distant, they are part of the care system.

8.4. The motivations for taking care of the sick relative

Caring for a sick loved one can be part of a triple action: give, receive and return. Giving your time, your affection, your attention, receiving in return a reward or even recognition. Since parents have given much before receiving it, there are "legitimate" and "continuous" expectations of help and support from their children (Godbout 2000).

The family duty, the strong parental bond with the sick person and the feeling of usefulness feed the motivation to take care of and bring help to the sick person. The obligation that is felt comes with blood ties and the moral principles of the family rejecting the idea that a "stranger" will come to take care of their close relative. This commitment corresponds to a legitimate duty. It reflects a social norm. For the majority of the interviews, the notion of obligation is most often expressed by the relatives of the sick as one of the values underlying the support. In the face of chronic illness, family ties become solid again from this logic of family duty, which makes it possible to temporarily disregard tensions and conflicts between family members.

> With us, a member of the family must take care of his or her close relative, especially the parents. It is quoted in the Koran that God insisted on caring for the parents and advised us not to frustrate them and not say hurtful words to them... I am relieved but may my mother rest in peace as I buried my mother after a great sacrifice... even when the members of the family quarrelled, the duty towards the patient reduces the conflicts between them...

Supporting a sick loved one is a duty and a debt. Family assistance is reactivated based on a logic of family duty, which is based on a gift-against-gift system and a sense of intergenerational obligation.

> When I was little and I fell ill, it was my father who cared for me, who looked after me, so it's my turn now to give him back his goodness and maybe if I have children, they are the ones who will take care of me later.

Children appear as actors at the heart of the patient support process. They mobilize around their relatives, often there is a helper who provides them with the necessary help for the management of the disease. For some, caring for close relatives relies on the availability of caregivers who will have to organize themselves to best manage difficult times and deal with their suffering. These caregivers believe that their support is a moral duty.

For some carers, it was the emotional ties at the start that most often motivated them to help or accompany a loved one, fed by a feeling of moral obligation towards their relative. Gratitude and duty also come to justify their commitment as the just return of a debt within the framework of conformity to the values of life.

The help given to the sick relative is also represented as a character of sacrifice. It is characterized by a strong valorization, for whom taking care of the sick parent is the sole reason for living. According to caregivers, they are, in fact, the only ones who can meet the needs and expectations of their close relatives. "That's the main thing for me, I can't do anything else while my father is suffering."

Caring for the sick is likened to a human act and an act of existence. The close relative can feel better by carrying out a human activity which is the fact of helping the other to feel like they exist.

8.5. The impact of care on the health of the patient's relative

Caring for a sick person can have physical, psychological and social consequences on the health of caregivers. In the management of the disease, caregivers are confronted with the physical and mental difficulty of care. If the loss of autonomy of a patient makes them vulnerable, the loved one who gradually compensates for the difficulties of this also finds themselves in a state of vulnerability. A very recurrent expression is: "The patient's relative becomes sicker than the sick person themself" or even "the person who takes care of a sick person is the real sick person."

The carers suffer from an internal wound. But they adapt to the constraints of the new reality and the family organization will be redefined. They take on tasks that quickly turn into morally painful experiences. They undergo a double penalty, that of forgetting their health and that of being forgotten. The health of family caregivers is often overlooked. Moral fatigue, stress, lack of time for oneself, isolation or the lack of recognition shown by the family circle are all the more often felt. Social disturbances are added when caregivers have a professional activity. It is difficult to reconcile the activity of supporting a loved one with the other aspects of their life. The commitment to take care of the sick loved one has serious consequences in terms of constraints and lack of availability to take care of oneself and one's health. For women, in particular, such a domestic and family working life leaves little room for professional activities and seems to prohibit a real professional career.

Doubt and ambivalence accompany the formulation of new life projects (building or buying a house, marriage, studies, professional projects, etc.). This seems to be at the root of feelings of failure, unfairness and guilt. Some caregivers admit that they are not living their own life to the full. Others have health issues themselves. They feel exhausted. The lives of carers are generally very difficult. It is from this sense of duty that carers can forget themselves and "neglect" their social and family life and their health. While this dedication comes naturally to them, it sometimes comes at the expense of their privacy and well-being as they are faced with responsibilities for which they are not always prepared. "For lack of means, listening and orientation, our task becomes heavy to bear... because the chronic disease itself is a source of stress and burden for the whole family".

If the help is initially related to an act of love concerning a sick parent, it is also marked by suffering, anxiety and depression. It seems that the person being helped and the helper must be at the center of care and health. In medical consultations, we often see that the caregiver is seeking care for their loved one, but they are not seeking care for themselves, while they too require more attention.

8.6. Conclusion

The role of patients' relatives has not always been obvious. Family help in caring for the sick tends to make them co-producers of the medical service and not mere companions. The care activities provided to the patient cannot be reduced to a predominantly medical approach or replace the shortcomings of the health system. Caring for people with chronic and long-term illnesses at home currently requires more attention to meet the emotional, relational and physical needs of the loved one. The recognition of them and their experiences in the different phases of the disease could change the world of medical institutions. It is even urged for the professionalization of care at home and to take care of the helper so that they can better take care of others.

8.7. References

Bachimot, J. (1998). "Les soins hospitaliers à domicile" entre démédicalisation hospitalière et médicalisation du domicile. In *L'ère de la médicalisation*, Pierre, A. and Daniel, D. (eds). Economica, Paris.

Baszanger, I. (1986). Les maladies chroniques et leur ordre négocié. *Revue française de sociologie*, 27(1), 3–27.

Beaud, S. and Weber, F. (2003). *Guide de l'enquête de terrain : produire et analyser des données ethnographiques*. La Découverte, Paris.

Benkada, H. and Mebtoul, M. (2018). Implication associative et travail de santé des personnes atteintes de sclérose en plaques et de leurs proches à Oran (Algérie). *Revue Insaniyat*, 80–81, 35–54 [Online]. Available at: http://journals.openedition.org/insaniyat/19117 [Accessed 10 January 2020].

Blanc, A. (ed.) (2010). Introduction. *Les aidants familiaux*. Grenoble University Press.

Bloch, M.A. (2012). Les aidants et l'émergence d'un nouveau champ de recherche interdisciplinaire. *Vie sociale*, 4, 11–29.

Cresson, G. (1993). Le travail de soins des mères de famille. In *L'enfant malade et le monde médical. Dialogue entre familles et soignants*, Cook, J. and Dommergues, J.-P. (eds). Syros, Paris.

Cresson, G. (2006), La production familiale de soins et de santé. La prise en compte tardive et inachevée d'une participation essentielle. *Recherches familiales*, 3, 6–15.

Cresson, G. and Mebtoul, M. (2010). *Famille et santé*. Editions ENSP, Rennes.

Godbout J.T. (2000). *Le don, la dette et l'identité*. La Decouverte, Paris.

Janzen, J.M. (1995). *La Quête de la thérapie au Bas-Zaïre*. Karthala, Paris.

Kane, H., Brignon, M., Kivits, J. (2018). Le rôle des proches de malades atteints d'un cancer : construction institutionnelle et expériences personnelles. In *Le cancer : un regard sociologique*, Ansellem, N. and Bataille, P. (eds). La Découverte, Paris.

Mebtoul, M. (2001). Les acteurs sociaux face à la santé publique : médecins, Etat et usagers. In *Systèmes et politiques de santé, de la santé publique à l'anthropologie*, Hours, B. (ed.). Karthala, Paris.

Mebtoul, M. (2005). *Médecins et patients en Algérie*. Editions Dar El Gharb, Oran.

Mebtoul, M. (2010). La dimension sociopolitique de la production de santé en Algérie. In *Famille et santé*, Cresson, G. and Mebtoul, M. (eds). Presses de l'EHESP, Rennes.

Mebtoul, M. and Tennci, L. (ed.) (2014). *Vivre le handicap et la maladie chronique. Les trajectoires des patients et des familles*. Editions GRAS, Oran.

Strauss, A. (1992). *La trame de la négociation, sociologie et interactionnisme, textes présentés par Baszanger*. L'Harmattan, Paris.

Waisman, R. (1995). Interactions familiales et impact de la technologie dans la gestion d'une maladie chronique chez l'enfant. *Sciences sociales et santé*, 13(1), 81–99.

9

Affective Dynamics of Caregivers to Those with Alzheimer's and Resilience. Self-(re)Construction through Two Devices: A Digital Platform and a Biographical Interview

One does not choose to be a caregiver. One becomes one, forced by the dependence of a loved one. The construction of this new identity that is imposed on the caregiver involves more or less public statements on what it represents in daily life, the gestures, the experienced emotions. Based on the hypothesis that the communication device has an influence on its conceptualization and on what the caregiver gives to see of this conceptualization, this chapter proposes to compare the affective dynamics of caregiving as expressed and constructed in 10 biographical semi-directive interviews (417,117 signs), extracted from the Accmadial corpus (*ACCompagnants des Malades Diagnostiqués d'Alzheimer*, led by PREFICS) and 10 discussions, extracted from the community forum dedicated to caregivers: *Aidons les nôtres* d'AG2R La Mondiale (144,006 signs). Impacted by the study of affects, feelings and emotions in several disciplinary fields and of the role of affects and of saying affects in particular (Damasio 2003, Averill and Rodis, in Barbier, Galatanu 1996), the comparison between the two devices highlights the singularity of each of the modalities but above all allows us to put forward several interpretative hypotheses concerning the construction of identity in caring in each of them.

Chapter written by Abdelhadi BELLACHHAB, Olga GALATANU and Valérie ROCHAIX.

9.1. Introduction

According to the results of the *OpinionWay* survey (2015), which discusses that, "Supporting a loved one who is losing their autonomy due to illness: motivations, experiences, aspirations"[1],

> long-term support for a loved one is not, as is often imagined, -[only] a compassionate approach, but a non-delegable moral commitment and an intimate experience of its own. This motivation is fueled by multiple feelings: a sense of family duty, a strong emotional bond with the sick person, a feeling of usefulness, and the fear that another person will take less good care of the loved one.

The caregiving relationship thus implies a moral commitment on the part of the caregiver mixed with hybrid, even sometimes contradictory, affective dynamics, oscillating between experiences of suffering and others of satisfaction, linked to the new caregiver role and its evolution from taking care "of the person" to "caring for the person"[2]. These dynamics participate in self-construction in this care relationship, where the latter is the space for a diversity of experiences and meanings that the caregiver associates with their situation. However, this self-construction is seen differently depending on the communication channel and the interpersonal device put in place. In this chapter, we will examine, on the one hand, the configuration of such affective relational dynamics, as well as their potential contribution to the feeling of resilience that the family caregiver could develop in the care relationship and, on the other hand, the way in which two identity-building devices participate in the (re)construction and unveiling of the affective experience of the family caregiver of a patient diagnosed with Alzheimer's. Since caregiving is an institution in the making, potentially constraining for these actors, in this case when it is a matter of caregivers displaying themselves emotionally, or even conforming, we hypothesize that these affective dynamics are doubly punctuated by hybrid axiological values: displaying both

---

1 Survey published on September 15, 2015, by the *Espace national de réflexion éthique sur les maladies neurodégénératives*.

2 Malherbe evokes these two stages in the evolution of the care relationship.

affective–volitive values characteristic of a "desire to help" and affective–ethical and moral (and deontic) values constituting a "duty to help". As a corollary, these dynamics vary in intensity, in nature (more volitional than deontic and vice versa) and in polarity (positive and/or negative affective) according to the self (re)construction device envisaged: the biographical interview or the discussion forum.

We organize our reflection in three stages. Firstly, we compare the two communication devices, and consequently the self-construction devices, in order to identify the specificities that are potentially incidental to the affective representations that family caregivers construct of themselves. We then introduce the theoretical and epistemological framework that constitutes our anchor for the definition of affects, in connection with feelings and emotions, and the classification of these with regard to the needs of this research. Finally, in a last part, subdivided into two subparts, we will analyze the expression of affects in the discussion forum, then in the semi-directive interview.

9.2. The biographical interview versus the discussion forum: two distinct devices of self-construction

Defining oneself in caregiving implies that one embodies a singular individual identity, but one that is at the same time embedded in a social identity that is constitutive of family caregivers. The institution (of caregiving) is made this way, without one necessarily recognizing oneself in it. One does not choose to be a caregiver, one becomes one. Identification with this institution takes place in different ways, among which we can mention the more or less public expression of family caregivers, through forums, discussion groups, blogs, sociological surveys, etc. These forums are places where caregivers can express their views and share their experiences. These forums are places for listening, expressing and sharing experiences of caregiving, an expression that varies according to the contexts, the interlocutors and the channels that participate in bringing it to light.

Divergence parameters	Discussion forum	Biographical interview
Intent to establish	Help and mutual aid (informational and emotional support)	Understanding the experience of caregiving through its expression (social recognition)
Speech initiated by...	The caregiver (Sometimes a facilitator)	The researcher
Speech constitution mode	Authentic speech	Solicited speech
Purpose of the exchange	Chosen theme	Fixed in advance by the researcher (part freedom)
Type of exchange	Polylogal	Dialogal
Mode of interaction	Online	Face to face
Channel and temporality	Written and asynchronous	Oral and synchronous
Interaction	Very present	Little present
Action time	More time for reflection/reaction/revision	Little time for reflection/reaction/revision
Participants	Caregivers, facilitator, geriatrician, "caregiver support" worker	Researcher + caregiver
Type of relation	Depending on the participants	Asymmetrical
Identity	Anonymous	Known

Table 9.1. *Aspects of divergence between the interview and the forum*

Whether they are soliciting or being solicited to speak, family caregivers do not have the same posture or the same attitudes with regard to their care relationship with their sick relatives: they express their emotional experience differently, they probably express the same experience, but conceptualized differently by profiling this or that facet of this experience. To support these postulates, we have chosen to focus on two distinct communication devices, in several respects. These are the semi-directive biographical interview adopted as part of the ACCMADIAL project[3] as a data collection tool with family caregivers of Alzheimer's patients in the Grand-Ouest region of France, and the forum of the community portal dedicated to caregivers, *Aidons les nôtres*, an AG2R La Mondiale site. Table 9.1 summarizes the main points of divergence between the two systems.

This comparison allows us to highlight the major differences in the reconstruction of a helping word and its availability within the institution of assistance, a word that is both a product of the actors of the institution and a constituent of it. The staging that each of the two devices proposes presages different discursive conceptualizations, with regard to divergent expectations and aspirations. In order to identify the specificities of the configuration and the construction of the affective experience that they offer, we take up each of these devices.

9.3. Spaces of expression

9.3.1. *The forum, constrained freedom and conventional authenticity?*

Our first sub-corpus is made up of excerpts from the *Aidons les nôtres* discussion forum, made available to family caregivers by the insurance company AG2R La Mondiale. This space declares a community of 6,000 caregivers who can:

> ask questions [online] and get answers from experts in 48 hours, find information thanks to more than 600 articles on all subjects (symptoms and pathologies, legal and financial, getting organized when you are a caregiver […] and exchange with other family caregivers.

---

3 The ACCMADIAL project (*ACCompagnants des Malades Diagnostiqués d'ALzheimer*), led by the PREFics laboratory (EA 7469, UBS), which includes our research, is studying the discourses of natural caregivers of patients diagnosed with Alzheimer's in order to describe their experiences and thus identify potential new ways of social recognition of "caregiving". It is currently financed by the IReSP within the framework of the call for projects Handicap et perte d'autonomie-session 10. It has also received broad financial and logistical support from the MSH Ange Guépin de Nantes and from the Université Bretagne Sud.

The corpus is made up of 10 discussions initiated either by a caregiver (a wife, 7 daughters, a son and a companion of a caregiver) or by the site moderator. A caregiver and a geriatrician were also involved.

The discussion forum, "automatically archived electronic correspondence, [...] a dynamic digital document, produced collectively in an interactive way" (Marcoccia 2004), is also considered as "the digital equivalent of sequences in the structural organization of a face-to-face conversation" (Kerbrat-Orecchioni 1990). Understood as a "hybrid device of mass interpersonal communication" (Baym 1998), it proposes written and asynchronous interactions, sometimes polylogal, sometimes dialogical and anonymized. In our case, a number of the speakers (moderator and speakers of the site) is identified in the exchanges. They practice one of the activities identified by Aguert et al. (2012), "[help and] mutual aid (informational and emotional support)". Faced with a difficult life situation, the support of a dependent relative, its users exploit this space to "share attitudes and affects" (Gauducheau 2008).

This corpus was chosen as a testimony of caregivers able to give an account of their self-representation and in the hypothesis, already formulated by Walther (1996, 2007), that its characteristics will favor expressive communication.

The sub-corpus *Aidons les nôtres* is distinguished (i) by its speech constitution mode (authentic discourse produced at the initiative of the caregiver, with a theme chosen by the caregiver and which expresses a need or in which they choose to insert), (ii) by intention of establishment (a speech to express a need) and (iii) by its asynchronous conversational form, polylogal and written.

However, the discussion forum, although it offers more freedom to speak than the interview, is still restrictive, either explicitly, if one looks at the "Charter of Participation", or implicitly, since the participant knows that they are speaking to experts (named as such by the site), in addition to other caregivers. So can we still talk about authenticity?

These characteristics lead us to make the following assumptions:

a) because anonymity makes the exposure of negative emotions less threatening (Caplan and Turner 2007), the discussion forum provides access to "authentic" feelings and emotions about the caregiving activity and relationship;

b) these feelings and emotions should be incidental to both the caregiver and the caregiver's interpretation of their action towards the patient;

c) their expressions could be enhancing for the caregiver and participate in the construction of a positive self-image justifying their activity as a caregiver, as well as devaluing for the other participants in the care of the dependency or for the person being cared for, the object of this care.

9.3.2. *The interview, a "position of social gaze"*

Our second sub-corpus consists of 10 semi-structured interviews. The caregivers were solicited by the researcher without having control over the established themes, although these were relatively less constraining as long as the caregiver's experience was relived narratively. The interviewer's interventions were limited as much as possible to the themes to be relived by the caregiver, to reminders or echoes.

The biographical interview, whose "objective is […] to elicit the production of words centered on the interviewee and giving an account of fragments of their existence, parts of their experience, moments in their life, elements of their situation" (Demazière 2008, p. 16), is thus a space conducive to the emotional unveiling and a moment of conceptualization of the interviewee's relationship with the self, with others and with the world. The family caregivers interviewed presented themselves by reconstructing their life trajectory, at least the one linked to the care relationship, a trajectory crossed by a number of displayed or induced identity dynamics. The caregivers retained a certain freedom within the constraints.

We have also postulated:

> that interviews with caregivers act as discursive training devices (DDs). These moments of existential self-training, like a form of "learning to be" (Carré 1997, p. 19), allow caregivers to have a certain social and institutional recognition of their singular, even novel but generalizable, knowledge of action, and consequently, of their new identity as caregivers (Bellachhab et al. 2022).

Unlike forums, at least in a more amplified way, these interviews established an asymmetrical relationship (Demazière 2008, p. 17). Present, from the outset, by the solicitation of the caregiver, it placed the researcher "in a position of social gaze" (ibid.). We suppose that this position of the researcher played, in the configuration provided by the interview and the identity construction that it enabled the caregiver, the role of the superego against which the latter reconstructed, measured and gauged implicitly or explicitly their words, acts, commitments and even disengagements. Faced with this position of social gaze, the caregiver sought to be recognized, not only for what they could do but also for what they indeed do, what they feel, with a view to meeting certain expectations, social norms or moral values.

In the same way as the forums, we argue that the interviews took part in this double game of valuing and devaluing on the part of the caregiver in relation to the actors of caregiving, if only in relation to the researcher opposite (and the institution they represent).

9.4. Theoretical and epistemological framework

Located at the crossroads of several disciplinary fields, our theoretical framework to approach the affects, feelings and emotions, is nourished by research in neurosciences (Damasio 2001, 2003), in psychology (Averill 1975, 1982, 1997, 1998; Plutchik 1980; Frijda 1986; Pagès 1986), philosophy (Spinoza 1993), psychology and communication sciences (Gauducheau 2008), education sciences, around the construction of identities and of course, language sciences

(Barbier and Galatanu 1998). In each of these disciplinary fields, the study of affects has led and still leads to the development of interfaces necessary to the elaboration of definitions and explanations of the mechanisms underlying their functioning. This is the case, for example, of neurosciences, which associate an interdisciplinary theoretical reflection (Damasio 1998) to experimental research (Damasio 1998; Adolphs et al. 2000; Plutchik 2002), to literary, linguistic and philosophical interrogations on the affective experience (Bertrand 1998). The work of the psychologist Robert Plutchik, for example, is finalized by the elaboration of a model, a "wheel of emotions" to account for motivating and nuanced emotions and to explain, among other things, phenomena that impact both individuals and society, such as suicide, violence and psychotherapies. In general, the work of psychologists, neuroscientists and philosophers is concerned with the links between emotions and language and/or languages and cultures.

More explicitly, Averill's work (1975, 1982, 1997) treats emotions in relation to the words that designate them and thus questions their origin, biological and social and cultural.

Moreover, the reflection on the (re)construction and identity dynamics of subjects in their interactions (Barbier and Galatanu 1998) takes up the question of the role of affects and of saying affects, present in Damasio as well as in Averill's work.

Without being able to dwell on the debates around the dichotomy of emotions versus feelings, we will propose an approach congruent with the linguistic analysis of the expression of affects in our corpora. Let us recall that these corpora "report" the affective experience of the carers and that of the patients, as it is apprehended by the carers. Our theoretical choices are justified first of all by this object, the labeling of affects, and by our objective, which is to give an account of the affective dynamics of the caregivers, in relation to their action of caregiving.

9.4.1. *Definitions of concepts: affects, emotions and feelings*

We can apprehend the affects as psychic experiences linked to the singularity of the situated experience.

Following James Averill's example, we understand emotions as different forms of experience, of psychic experience, belonging to a "family resemblance", in the sense of Wittgenstein (1953). For Averill, as for other researchers, notably in linguistics (Wierzbicka 1992), even if emotions vary from one culture to another, they fulfill three prototypical conditions forming a family resemblance (Fehr and Russell 1984; Shaver et al. 1987; Averill 1997): passivity, intentionality and subjectivity.

Passivity

In linguistic terms, passivity refers to the semantic-syntactic role of the subject experiencing the emotion (Fillmore 1977).

However, when the caregiver's discourse evokes the emotion that their action as caregiver provokes in the patient, the latter appears most often in the object position (objective case in Fillmore's terminology). In other words, we note a semantic-syntactic recategorization of the experiential dative into the experiential objective and this especially when the phases of the illness transform the early supportive care into existential care and finally into ontological care (Malherbe 2015, 2019a).

> Although it is no longer common to speak of emotions as passions, the connotation of passivity (of being "overcome") is implicit in emotional concepts. We "fall" in love, are "gripped" by anger, "can't help" but hope, and so forth. Because emotional concepts connote passivity, emotions themselves have often been likened to reflexes and simple sensory experiences, which are also beyond personal control. As will be discussed below, however, people typically have more control over their

emotions than the connotation of passivity would suggest (Averill 1997, p. 514).

Intentionality

Emotions are intentional in the sense described by Searle (1983), i.e. they are referred to something: an emotionally competent stimulus (Damasio 2003), object, situation, human being, etc. This distinguishes them from simple reflexes, which Damasio calls background emotions.

Subjectivity

While discussing and questioning the subjective/objective dichotomy, Averill insists that emotions are subjective in the sense that they are an attribute of the subjective extreme of experience.

This focus on the experimenter and not on the object that constitutes the emotionally competent stimulus is interesting linguistically since it participates in the subjectivation of the discourse. The analysis of affective dynamics is thus based on the linguistic marks of this position-taking, of this break in indifference (Lavelle 1991) and joins the analysis of modalities.

To understand the notion of feeling and to position it in the field of affects, we can resort to the concept of construction of a conceptual and semantic representation of a psychic experience. This cognitive and discursive construction implies the recognition of this experience "as belonging to a set of known and socially shared experiences, which gives it a lasting and less singular character" (Barbier and Galatanu 1998, p. 48). Pagès (1986) speaks of an association of this psychic state with an inner discourse that names both the object and the nature of the relationship.

9.4.2. *Classes of emotions*

There are many proposals for classifying and organizing the semio-sphere of affects, in this case emotions. However, for our study, we retain only three elements linked to the status of the caregiver:

a) The distinction proposed by Damasio (2003, pp. 51–52), between primary emotions and social emotions.

The first, basic emotions, such as fear, anger, disgust, surprise, sadness and happiness, correspond, according to us, philosophically to thin concepts (Williams 1985; Putnam 2002), organized on the positive–negative axis, the second, which integrate primary emotions, correspond to thick affective concepts, the thin values being incidental to others: sympathy, embarrassment, shame, guilt, pride, envy, gratitude, admiration, indignation, contempt. They are also organized around the positive and negative extremes.

In the study of the caregiver's identity dynamics, as it appears in the two types of discourse present in our corpus, these two classes of emotions characterize the singular experience they have in their new status, for the first, and their family and social status for the second.

b) The organization of emotions on the positive–negative axis, whether they are primary or social emotions.

c) A certain direction of fit of the emotion and the object that triggered it (the emotionally competent stimulus).

In terms of the lexicalization of these concepts, we can speak of designations promoting the influence of the subject experimenter of the emotion on the world, on the transformation of the world (e.g. the desire) and of designations promoting the influence of the context, in particular of the emotionally competent stimulus on the experimenter subject (sadness, sorrow, grief). It must be recognized that in French, and probably in many other languages, it is difficult to find emotions whose direction of fit corresponds to the first case. On the other hand, the semantic analysis of the designations of social emotions reveals affordances of action, decision-making, intervention and, consequently, of a willingness to assume the status of helper.

The triangulation of these three elements leads us to put forward a hypothesis that we will have to validate with the analysis of our corpus. We believe that negative social emotions, such as guilt and shame, are associated with the awareness of a duty to assume the caregiver status, despite the many primary, basic, negative emotions that accompany this status. The corollary of this hypothesis is that the feeling of positive social emotions, such as compassion and gratitude, is associated with the desire, or even the will, to assume the caregiver status, and that positive basic emotions also accompany acting in accordance with this status.

9.5. The emotional experience of caregivers through two communication devices

9.5.1. *Tool-based approach to the corpus*

We chose in this analysis to focus on the expression of affective experience through the words that designate it in the two aforementioned devices. Our research was therefore limited to "said emotions", according to Micheli's terminology (2014). For an initial exploratory approach, we decided to limit ourselves to a portion of the ACCMADIAL corpus (interviews) and a single discussion forum for the helping public. From the 108 interviews[4] obtained, we retained 10 interviews for this study, with the concern of respecting a certain heterogeneity guaranteeing as much as possible a certain representativeness of the interviewed public; on the other hand, for the forums, we did not have control over the participants. The choice of discussions was determined by three criteria: the first, and most important, was the link with specific help for patients diagnosed with Alzheimer's; the second was the number of interventions in the discussion; and finally the number of views of the discussion. Table 9.2 shows some statistical data on the participants in each device and the number of signs in each corpus.

In view of the size of the two corpora, a first approach was necessary to identify the words that designate the experienced affects.

---

4 Including 27 interviews conducted with the same caregivers on two, three or four occasions, at least six months apart. The transcriptions were completed by Solenne Latil, Emmanuelle Vade and Bérangère Bouteille. We would like to thank them.

A first identification was carried out from the determination of the reference universes by the Tropes software. These universes contain "the very significant nouns [of the] text and certain proper nouns" (Tropes manual, [Online] (2021)).

Relationship with the person being cared for	Interview corpus	Corpus forum[5]
Spouse	2	-
Wife	4	1
Partner	1	-
Sister	1	-
Daughter	2	7
Son	-	1
Carer's carer	-	1
Total	10	10
Number of signs	417,117	144,006

Table 9.2. *Composition of the study sample*

This lexical retrieval was completed by a manual analysis of the full lexical table established with the Lexico5 software, from which the extracts in context were obtained using the concordancer. We retained and therefore added a nominal form (solitude) and adjectival forms associated with the words of the first list such as happy and pleasant.

We have organized the identified lexicalized affects in Table 9.3, distinguishing primary emotions from secondary emotions and those incidental to the caregiver or the caregiver's action towards the sick person according to the caregiver themselves.

5 Only the initiators of the discussion were taken into account for the forum.

Emotions	Incidents involving	Accmadial interviews	Discussion forum
Primary	The caregiver	Fear (16.5%)	Fear (33.3%)
		No desire (16.5%)	Sadness (19.4%)
		Worry (11.65%)	Anxiety (13.8%)
		Concern (7.76%)	Sorrow (13.8%)
		Suffering (5.82%)	Grief (11.1%)
		Horror (5.82%)	Pain (5.5%)
		Stress (3.88%)	
		Sadness (2.91%)	
		Panic (1.94%)	
		Pain (0.97%)	
		Annoyance (0.97%)	
		Despair (0.97%)	
		Disappointment (0.97%)	
		The jitters (0.97%)	
		Feeling wanted by the patient + (4.85%)	(Only) joy (2.8%)
		Pleasure (3.88%)	
		Love (3.88%)	
		Contentedness (3.88%)	
		Relief (2.91%)	
		Happiness (0.97%)	
		Joy (0.97%)	
	The patient	Worries (27.27%)	Happiness (57.1%)
		Suffering (18.18%)	Pleasure (35.71%)
		Stress (18.18%)	(Small) joys (7.1%)
		Concern (9.09%)	
		Pain (9.09%)	
		Content (18.18%)	
Social	The caregiver	Guilt	Guilt (66.6%)
			Envy (11.1%)
			Regret (11.1%)
			Compassion (4.2%)
			Tenderness (7%)
	The patient	(Have) fun (64%)	Relief
		Relief (36%)	

Table 9.3. *Inventory of lexicalized affects in the two devices*

A global overview of this affective configuration in the two devices allows us to draw some preliminary conclusions:

– The affective palette in the interviews is richer than that of the forum (with shared emotions), but this richness must be put into perspective in view of the vocation of the two devices (the interview solicits the lived experience in a certain exhaustiveness where the caregiver is invited, by the very communication contract of the interview, to come back to the care relationship; the forum welcomes a punctual polylogal speech), the size of the two corpora (the corpus of the interviews is almost three times as large as the corpus of the forum).

– Emotions incidental to the caregiver are more present in both corpora, and rather negative, contrary to those incidental to the patient, which when they are related to the action of the caregiver are positive in the forum, but positive and negative in the interviews.

– Primary emotions are clearly more present than social emotions.

– In the forum, the caregivers express positive and negative social emotions incidental to the two care partners, while in the interviews, they express negative emotions incidental to the caregiver, but positive emotions incidental to the care receiver.

The strong presence of negative affects, as illustrated in Table 9.3, confirms the doubly trying, even painful experience of caregiving, which places the caregiver "[...] between the societal imposition (having to take care of a dependent loved one for moral and pragmatic reasons) and the ability [...] to cope with this imposition". (Garric et al. 2020). This paradoxical injunction can be seen through a relational dynamic fluctuating between acceptance and rejection of this new function status, between *having to* assume it and *willing to* assume it. Caregiving as a relationship of care (and of taking care) thus presupposes a moral commitment on the part of the caregiver mixed with hybrid, even sometimes contradictory, affective dynamics, oscillating between experiences of fear, anxiety, sadness and pain, and others of love, pleasure and joy, linked to the new caregiver role and its evolution from taking care "of the person" to "caring for the person". Because of their new status, caregivers find themselves having to manage a situation where the unpleasant is often joined to the useful, even the necessary, nevertheless the pleasant is not completely absent.

The experience of caregiving a priori as a "burden"[6] suggests that there are more negative affects associated with this ordeal and with the evolution of caregiving, from the first day of the diagnosis to the eventual taking into care, of the person being cared for, in a care home or until their death. However, the inventory of lexicalized affects reported by the caregiver in interviews as well as in the forum, whether these affects are incidental to the caregiver or to the person being cared for, allows us to glimpse these moments of shared pleasure, of love, as well as and above all, desires to do good for the patient. This configuration supports the idea of an apparent malaise of the caregiver, but allows these positive emotions to emerge against the background of a frustrating and painful experience. This positive dimension of the affects is revealed more in the interviews than in the forum, and is more apparent to the caregiver than to the person being cared for in the interviews, and vice versa.

Having highlighted these similarities and divergences between the expression of affects in the two devices, we will formulate interpretative hypotheses regarding the construction of affective identity in the assistance that each of the two corpora proposes. Finally, we will illustrate these affects with one frequent emotion that is common to both corpora and another that is different.

9.5.2. *The emotional experience reconstructed lexically in the forum*

The fourth reference universe identified after those of health, family (208 items each) and time (124), that of feelings counts 110 occurrences of 41 nouns, the most frequent words being *friend(s)* and *partner*, followed by *affects*, *fear*, *relief* and *guilt*, without taking into

6 "The dominant literature on family assistance and caregiver support focuses on caregiver burden. [...] Family caregiving is conceptualized, with reference to stress-coping theory, as a major stress that the caregiver must combat by implementing 'good' strategies" (Coudin and Mollard 2011).

account the turns of speech. After having excluded the words designating family and friendly relationships (such as *friend*, *boyfriend*, *partner*, etc.), we retained from this universe the words: *sadness*, *sorrow* and *grief*; *pleasure* and *joy*, *happy*, *fear*, *anxiety*, *relief*, *pain* as well as *compassion*, *tenderness*, *guilt* and *regret*. Taking into account the verbal or adjectival forms of these words, guilt is in first place in this ranking with 18 occurrences, far ahead of fear and sadness.

A reading of this corpus reveals a first specificity in the distinction between primary emotions and social emotions when these are incidental to the caregiver. The caregivers display as many primary emotions as social ones, unlike the caregivers in the interviews. In a space of help and mutual aid such as the forum, where experts and caregivers rub shoulders, we can expect, on the part of the family caregivers, a characterization of the affective experience in its social dimension as well as in its primary dimension more oriented towards oneself, implicitly taking a position in relation to the weight of ethical/moral values mixed with the expressed affects, as in the case of guilt, regret or compassion and relief.

This social dimension of emotions is accompanied by an accentuation of the basic positive affects of the person being cared for, while the primary positive affects of the caregiver are almost absent or erased. We can hypothesize here that there is a focus on sacrificial care, where the caregiver, by the nature of the communication device used, emphasizes what they do for the person being cared for while questioning the sufficiency of the help provided, without forgetting the trying experience of caregiving.

The rules for the confidentiality of data extracted from discussion forums do not allow us to quote extracts; we can however highlight several mechanisms:

– the convocation of positive values in connection with the action of the caregiver; it is manifested on the one hand in the lexicon (pleasure, joy, happy) in constructions such as:

Caregiver says he saw his mother (who is being cared for) "happy" BECAUSE of Christmas with the family.

Caregiver says he looks for ways to make his mother's life "happy".

– the unidirectionality of the exchange is accessible through syntactic clues; for all *pleasure* convocations, the helper is the agent and the helper is the beneficiary, while in the case of *neg_pleasure*, the helper is the beneficiary;

– the stressful nature is seen especially through the *fear* expressed by the caregiver, especially a prospective fear, followed by a verbal form. In the statements including the word *fear*, we note for the experimenting caregiver, sequences such as:

- *fear* + *verbal* phrase, about the quality of the help, the quality of the caregiver or the impact of the help on the caregiver's life.

In the statements placing the helped as experimenter, it appears such as:

– *fear* + *noun phrase*, relating to the caregiver's social or natural environment (fear of the dark, children, etc.).

Guilt is very present in the corpus, with 18 occurrences of the word in a nominal or verbal form.

In the caregiver's words, guilt is stated or feared. Asserted, the guilt is possibly followed by an adverb and sometimes by a connector that weakens the argument. The statements produced are such as:

– *I + feel guilty (a little) YET [unable to continue, at the end of my tether).*

- *[+ need for respite];*

- *[+ explanation of the supportive actions].*

Guilt is an emotion/feeling introduced and rejected in exchanges with other participants, with imperative or imperative infinitive forms ("do not feel guilty", "no guilt") or the performative verb "forbid" ("I forbid you to feel guilt").

Relief[7] is present in the corpus but in the discourse of other participants. The interlocutor caregiver or the caregiver in question is the beneficiary. It is the caregiver who needs to be relieved, not the one who relieves, or the one who is relieved.

In this corpus, the caregiver constructs a relatively positive image of their action, as is the case in the Accmadial corpus. On the other hand, they express more concern about the personal cost of their involvement, as shown by the constructions with *fear of.* This explicitness is not, however, condemned by the other participants, who use *neg_guilt* several times and say that they need to be relieved of the burden of caring.

The linguistic and discursive analysis of the forum corpus also sheds light on the link between motivation in the action of helping and affects such as the duty to help or the imposition of helping. This link is a theme developed in the exchanges.

It is questioned by the caregivers of their parents with an argument such as:

– *Caregiver emotional values (love/affective/compassion);*

– *Ethical and moral values (loyalty/benevolence/debt/fear of being inadequate);*

– *Deontic values (duty).*

– *It is also raised by the intervening professionals, then constructed such as:*

- *Helping = Ethical and emotional value BUT MUST NOT "structure" the assistance/*

This construction is based on repetitions and sequences of discordant arguments between the caregiver about themselves and the

---

7 Relief of sorrow, a moral or psychological pain in someone: the relief of miseries; impression felt at the disappearance of a difficulty, an inconvenience, an anxiety. E.g. "It is a relief to know they have arrived" (Larousse).

caregiver about caregivers (in general). We also note here arguments differentiated according to the age of the caregivers. While the right to respite is often linked to the fact of being able to carry out one's role as a carer (an argument in favor of caring), it is linked to the right to protect oneself and in opposition to the construction of the "sacrificial figure" when it is a young carer. The argument is then developed in favor of the caregiver as an individual.

9.5.3. *The emotional experience reconstructed lexically in the interviews*

After filtering words denoting family and friendship relationships into the reference universe of feelings, we identified 30 lexicalized affects with 103 occurrences. Three-quarters of the primary emotions incident to the caregiver are negative, and one-quarter positive. Proportionally to the total number of affects incident to the helped, almost the same distribution applies.

As mentioned above, the experience of help is one of suffering, pain and especially fear.

> 1) Yvonne: ah well what **frightened** me, it was his behavior that was, uh he was losing his balance [acq] he was no longer there.

> 2) Romane: well I don't know, uh, I was **afraid** of hurting him.

> 3) Romane: […] and then finally at the beginning I was **afraid** that it would disturb him/his intimacy it's still embarrassing, eh [acq] eh at the beginning when I accompanied him to the toilet.

> 4) Romane: […] I was **afraid** that he would do something about it and that you shouldn't act urgently, you shouldn't, you shouldn't be in a hurry, even if it is urgent.

The "horrible" and "painful" experience of caregiving, more widespread in the literature under the name of "burden", is confirmed in this corpus through a diversity of negative affects, dominated by *fear* for oneself (of the sick person, of the future, etc.) and for the sick person (fear of hurting them, of disturbing them, of seeing them take the wheel, etc.), and declined in suffering, passing through emotions of worry, sadness, disappointment, despair, etc.

Nevertheless, moments of joy and happiness are always present, much more than in the forum. The following example illustrates this dichotomy between burden and joy.

> 5) Flore: […] for me it's normal it's not a burden and it's a **joy** to see that everything I do that she listens to me already that uh that she uh that she has confidence in me in what I advise her to do…

Pleasure (often shared), whether in its primary dimension (having fun) or social dimension (giving pleasure), supports this joy, by being first incidental to the caregiver and then to the person being cared for.

> 6) Richard: […] well, it's the books that are there but I still want them [e] I take them out, it gives me **pleasure** to touch them, even though I fly through them, it's arti-(x) it's artificial perhaps but I've read some, some I've read quite a few…

> 7) Félicie: […] to make sure that he is well, I want him to be well, to **please** him with meals.

This positive affective interlude reminds us, to a certain extent, of helper-satisfaction (Caradec 2009), associated precisely with an experience of satisfaction (to moments of happiness) by the caregiver, which would counterbalance the ordeal of caregiving. The interviews reveal a panoply of contradictory experiences of caregiving because, as Caradec (2009, p. 113) states, "constraints and satisfactions can be intertwined in the same interview and there are different ways of 'living well' and 'living badly' in regards to the situation". Are we dealing here with what is called in social psychology a cognitive dissonance suggested by this tension between "having to help", symptomatic of the moral societal imposition, and "willing to help" implying the freedom to "be able to do" and "not to do"?

We suggest that caregiving is a tug-of-war between the awareness of the duty to help as an ethically imposed burden, underpinned by a significant negative affective charge, and the desire/willingness to do so, sprinkled with positive affective intervals. This positive aspect of the affective relationship that emerges within the painful experience of caregiving would serve, for the caregiver, as an outlet to (self-) justify a limitless commitment or better, to find a balance between the weight of *having* to help one's spouse/father/mother, etc. and the joy or pleasure of *willing* to help. Experiencing and recounting these moments of happiness and the resulting affects reflect a rebalancing between this weight of duty and this consolation of desire. It is therefore a question of interweaving the affective experience of moral duty and the affective experience of the will and desire to do of the caregiver.

Surprisingly, this tension is not accompanied, as we might expect, by a strong feeling of guilt. Unlike the caregivers in the forum, the only two occurrences concern putting the sick person in a care home.

> 8) Caregiver: well, we always **feel** a little **guilty** when we introduce the people [to the care home].

> 9) Félicie: [...] but when I went I saw on her face that she was beaming to see me and that's when I **feel guilty** and I say to myself: well if in fact uh I should go more often, because I don't go during the week with my work schedule and she goes in the evening at 5:00 pm.

Is this absence linked to the communication contract between the researcher and the caregiver? Precisely, in connection with the position of social gaze associated with the researcher, we can hypothesize that it is thanks to this desire to see the positive side of the helping relationship (or to confirm it) that the family caregiver refuses to feel guilty in the face of the presupposed ethical/moral gaze of the interviewer, except in the case of the transfer of the sick person to a care home. These moments of pleasure that they share with their sick relative, where they "relieve" them (example 10), are moments of satisfaction with their action.

> 10) Yvonne: [...] with his doctor in [ent=municipality] who sent prescriptions with what I described to the pharmacy in [ent=commune] so that I could make the, to succeed in **relieving** him of pain and things like that.

9.6. Conclusion

The two communication devices, the interview as well as the forum, offer us each in its own way two different affective scenarios, crossed by a diverse palette and relational dynamics of a weak actor. These scenarios seem to fit the specificities of the discursive space offered by the two devices.

The affective dynamics involved in these scenarios, which contribute to the construction and affirmation of identity, combined with their action tendencies, in this case that of the positive approach, would constitute a strong motive in the eyes of family caregivers to pursue their mission. Example 11 illustrates a certain superiority of the emotional bond (my husband) over the moral bond of having to help the other person.

> 11) Gertrude: [...] sometimes I say to myself "but I'm going to hold on, yes" well yes, I think it's still my husband and I have to help him, we have to move forward together and we have to get to the point where he'll really be well, he'll be too affected, no doubt physically, because it'll happen unfortunately.

Although minimal, the positive emotional experience generates a form of resilience in family caregivers by leading them to take care of their sick loved ones until the end, often to the detriment of their health, or even their lives.

9.7. References

Adolphs, R., Damasio, H., Tranel, D., Cooper, G., Damasio, A.R. (2000). A role of somatosensory cortices in the visual recognition of emotion as revealed by three-dimensional lesion mapping. *The Journal of Neuroscience*, 20, 2683–2690.

Aguert, M., Marcoccia, M., Atifi, H., Gauducheau, N., Laval, V. (2012). La communication expressive dans les forums de discussion : émotions et attitude ironique chez l'adolescent. *Tranel*, 57, 63–82.

Averill, J.R. (1975). A semantic atlas of emotional concepts. *JSAS Catalog of Selected Documents in Psychology*, 330(5), 513–541.

Averill, J.R. (1982). *Anger and Aggression: An Essay on Emotion*. Springer-Verlag, New York.

Averill, J.R. (1997). The emotions. An integrative approach. In *Handbook of Personality Psychology*, Hogan, R., Johnson, J., Briggs, S. (eds). Academic Press, London.

Averill, J.P. and Rodis, P.T. (1996). Le rôle du langage dans les transformations émotionnelles. In *Action, affects et transformation de soi*, Barbier, J.M. and Galatanu, O. (eds). PUF, Paris.

Barbier, J.M. and Galatanu, O. (1998). De quelques liens entre action, affects et transformation de soi. In *Action, affects et transformation de soi*, Barbier, J.M. and Galatanu, O. (eds). PUF, Paris.

Baym, N.K. (1998). The emergence of the on-line community. In *Cybersociety 2.0: Revisiting Computer-Mediated Communication and Community*, Jones S.G. (ed.). Sage, Thousand Oaks.

Bellachhab, A., Galatanu, O., Le Gal, S. (2022). La fonction formative des dispositifs discursifs de recueil de données : les savoirs d'action des aidants de malades diagnostiqués d'Alzheimer. *Chemins de formation*, L'Harmattan, Paris.

Bertrand, D. (1998). De l'action à la passion : les variations sémiotiques de l'identité. In *Action, affects et transformation de soi*, Barbier, J.M. and Galatanu, O. (eds). PUF, Paris.

Blanchet, A. (1991). L'interactivité des relances dans l'entretien d'enquête. *Connexions*, 57(1), 38–67.

Caplan, S. and Turner, J. (2007). Bringing theory to research on computer-mediated comforting communication. *Computers in Human Behavior*, 23(2), 985–998.

Caradec, V. (2009). Vieillir, un fardeau pour les proches ? *Lien social et politiques*, 62, 111–122.

Carre, P. (1997). La galaxie de l'autoformation aujourd'hui. In *L'autoformation : psychopédagogie, ingénierie et sociologie*, Carre, P., Moisan, A., Poisson, D. (eds). PUF, Paris.

Coudin, G. and Mollard, J. (2011). Difficultés, stratégies de faire face et gratifications : première étape de validation du CADI-CAMI-CASI auprès d'un échantillon français d'aidants familiaux. *Gériatrie et psychologie neuropsychiatrie du vieillissement*, 93, 363–378.

Cyrulnik, B. and Seron, C. (eds) (2004). *La résilience ou comment renaître de sa souffrance*. Fabert, Paris.

Damasio, A. (1998). The human amygdala in social judgement. *Nature*, 393, 470–474.

Damasio, A. (2001). *L'erreur de Descartes*. Odile Jacob, Paris.

Damasio, A. (2003). *Spinoza avait raison. Joie, tristesse, le cerveau des émotions*. Odile Jacob, Paris.

Demaziere, D. (2008). L'entretien biographique comme interaction négociations, contre-interprétations, ajustements de sens. *Langage et société*, 123(1), 15–35.

Fehr, B. and Russell, J.A. (1984). Concept of emotion viewed from a prototype perspective. *Journal of Experimental Psychology: General*, 113, 464–486.

Fillmore, C. (1997). The case for case reopened. In *Grammatical Relations*, Cole, P. and Sadock, J.M. (eds). Academic Press, New York.

Frijda, N.H. (1986). *The Emotions*. Cambridge University Press, Cambridge.

Galatanu, O. (2000). Langue, discours et système de valeurs. In *Curiosité linguistiques*, Suomela-Salmi, E. (ed.). Presses Universitaires de Turku.

Galatanu, O. (2018). *La sémantique des possibles argumentatifs : génération et (re)construction discursive du sens linguistique*. Peter Lang, Brussels.

Garric, N., Pugnière-Saavedra, F., Rochaix, V. (2020). Construction langagière de la figure de l'aidant du malade d'Alzheimer : dénominations et mise en mots interdiscursive dans les pratiques. *CORELA – COgnition, REprésentation, LAngage*, 18–1 [Online] Available at: http://journals.openedition.org/corela/11302.

Gauducheau, N. (2008). La communication des émotions dans les échanges médiatisés par ordinateur : bilan et perspectives. *Bulletin de psychologie*, 496(4), 389–404.

Kerbrat-Orecchioni, C. (1990). *Les interactions verbales*, volume I. Armand Colin, Paris.

Lavelle, L. (1991). *Traité des valeurs I : Théorie générale de la valeur*. Presses Universitaires de France, Paris.

Malherbe, M. (2015). *Alzheimer. La vie, la mort, la reconnaissance*. Vrin, Paris.

Malherbe, M. (2019a). *Alzheimer. De l'humanité des hommes*. Vrin, Paris.

Malherbe, M. (2019b). Le soin de reconnaissance : Alzheimer. In *Philosophie du soin. Santé, autonomie, devoirs*, Durand, G. and Dabouis, G. (eds). Vrin, Paris.

Maroccia, M. (2004). L'analyse conversationnelle des forums de discussion : questionnements méthodologiques. *Les Carnets du CEDISCOR*, 8, 23–38.

Micheli, R. (2014). *Les émotions dans les discours. Modèle d'analyse, perspectives empiriques*. De Boeck Supérieur, Louvain-la-Neuve.

Pages, M. (1986). *Trace ou sens, le système émotionnel*. Hommes et groupes, Paris.

Philippot, P. (1997). Schèmes cognitifs et expérience émotionnelle : le cas des sensations corporelles. In *La psychologie sociale. Tome III : L'ère de la cognition*, Leyens, J.P. and Beauvois, J.L. (eds). Presses Universitaires de Grenoble, Grenoble.

Plutchik, R. (1980). *Emotion: A Psychoevolutionary Synthesis*. Harper & Row, New York.

Plutchik, R. (2002). *Emotions and Life: Perspectives from Psychology, Biology, and Evolution*. American Psychological Association, Massachusetts.

Putnam, H. (2002). *Fait/valeur, la fin d'un dogme et autres essais*, translated by Caveribere, M. and Cometti, J.-P. Éditions de l'Éclat, Paris.

Searle, J.R. (1983). *Intentionality. An Essay in the Philosophy of Mind.* Cambridge University Press, Cambridge.

Searle, J.R. (2010). *Making the Social World: The Structure of Human Civilization.* Oxford University Press, New York.

Shaver, P., Schwartz, J., Kirson, D., O'Connor, C. (1987). Emotion knowledge: Further exploration of a prototype approach. *Journal of Personality and Social Psychology*, 52, 1061–1086.

Solomon, R.C. (1993). *The Passions: Emotions and the Meaning of Life.* Hackett, Indiapolis.

Spinoza, B. (1993). *Ethique*, translated by Appuhn, C. Flammarion, Paris.

Walther, J.B. (1996). Computer-mediated communication: Impersonal, interpersonal and hyperpersonal interaction. *Communication Research*, 23(1), 3–43.

Walther, J.B. (2007). Selective self-presentation in computer-mediated communication: Hyperpersonal dimensions of technology, language, and cognition. *Computers in Human Behaviors*, 23(5), 2538–2557.

Wierzbicka, A. (1992). Defining emotion concepts. *Cognitive Science*, 16, 539–581.

Williams, B. (1985). *Ethics and the Limits of Philosophy.* Harvard University Press, Cambridge, MA.

Wittgenstein, L. (1953). *Philosophical Investigations.* Basil Blackwell & Mott, Oxford.

10

Co-constructing a Territory that Provides Assistance

Carers provide free assistance to relatives who are dependent on them for the activities of daily living. This act of assistance entails multiple evolving needs for the carers. Public policies in France have taken up this major social and societal challenge by developing a national plan for old age and loss of autonomy, in which support for carers is promoted. At the same time, they are prioritizing the maintenance of dependent people at home in order to rethink the care pathway and the quality of life of people losing their independence. In this context, carers are at the heart of the mutual aid system. It is from this observation that the "By and for carers" action carried out by DanaeCare was born in 2019. Developed in a health democracy as an inclusive and transpathological approach, the action mobilized the associative, academic and institutional actors of the Loire region in order to fulfill the needs of local carers, design adapted solutions with them and for them and document the whole system. The aim of the whole action is thus to co-construct a territory that helps carers. After a year of consultation, during which participatory research tools were mobilized, the action raised several issues relating to care and is now leading to a federative project: the Carers' Stopover.

10.1. Introduction

Since 2019, the association DanaeCare has been leading an action aimed at co-constructing a territory for caregivers in Saint-Etienne,

Chapter written by André SIMONNET, Julia GUDEFIN and Maya CHABANE.

France[1]. Through this action, DanaeCare is interested in the figure of the caregiver, the "shadow" or "invisible associate" of the patient in their care journey, as may have been said when referring to caregivers (Rossinot 2019).

To approach the figure of the caregiver, it is necessary to understand how the notion is defined. We need to "understand" because this notion is subject to different definitions and qualifiers depending on the quality of the person being helped (a person with a disability or a person in a situation of dependence/loss of autonomy).

In any case, whether they are qualified as "family caregivers", "close caregivers" or "natural caregivers", caregivers – whatever their qualification – provide free assistance to a person within their entourage who is dependent on them for the activities of daily life, whether it be material, financial, administrative, psychological or moral support. This is how the European Charter for Family Caregivers or the French legislation[2] defines the family caregiver or the close caregiver. A parent, child, spouse, neighbor or friend becomes a "caregiver" as soon as an act of assistance is performed, on a regular basis, whether permanent or not, for a person around them who is disabled and/or dependent due to age or not.

The concept of caregiving does not only represent the caregiver and the patient. It represents above all the relationship between them and the ecosystem in which this relationship is embedded. Thus, caregiving covers both the form and means of assistance and the

---

1 Founded in 2012 and located in Saint-Étienne, the association DanaeCare helps users, actors and institutions of healthcare to promote the human at the heart of care. See: danaecare.com.

2 "Is considered as a close caregiver of an elderly person, their spouse, the partner with whom they have entered into a civil solidarity pact or their cohabitant, a parent or an ally, defined as family caregivers, or a person residing with them or maintaining close and stable ties with them, who helps them, on a regular and frequent basis, in a non-professional capacity, to perform all or part of the acts or activities of daily life" (art. 51 of law no. 2015-1776 of December 28, 2015, for the adaptation of society to aging, *JO* of December 29, 2015, codified in art. L. 113-1-3 of the Social Action and Family Code).

different actors involved in this relationship (care professionals, social workers, etc.)[3]. In this way, this concept encompasses all the organization and resources, human and material, mobilized by the helping relationship. As a result, caregiving is becoming a real public health issue.

Based on this observation, the approach initiated by DanaeCare "co-constructing a territory that helps caregivers" focuses on the caregivers of people affected by all pathologies – from old age to mental health – and on their pathway in the ecosystem of care at the scale of a given territory: the Loire department and, more specifically, Saint-Etienne.

This approach was based on several approaches. First, it is a territorial approach that defines the action for caregivers. Historically in France, the subject and status of caregivers have been built around old age and loss of autonomy. This has resulted in a territorial translation of the caregiving ecosystem segmented by major themes or pathologies: old age and loss of autonomy, physical disability/illness and mental disability. It has become apparent that this segmentation complicates the pathways of caregivers whose loved ones are sometimes at the intersection of pathologies. Hence, the project carried out by DanaeCare was constructed in an interdisciplinary and transpathological way in order to propose a coherent territorial approach for caregivers and caregivers' actors.

Second, a legal approach is essential to understanding legislation. As the legislative and regulatory provisions relating to caregivers are disparate, recourse to the law is all the more difficult for caregivers. Whether it is a question of their status or their role in the care of their loved one[4], the situation of caregivers and their trajectory in the ecosystem of care are complicated by the disparity of texts and legal

3 Bergua, B. and Bouisson, J. (eds) (2021). *Aidons les aidants, osons l'Aidance.* Editions In Press, Paris.

4 Family caregivers are often associated with the "trusted person" who constitutes a legal status that is identified and supervised in the hospitalization process of a loved one.

statuses relating to caregivers (close caregiver, family caregiver, natural caregiver).

Then, the caregiving relationship is identified through the prism of a sociological approach. Based on the 2017 report of the Caisse Nationale de Solidarité pour l'Autonomie (CNSA) entitled "*Accompagnement des proches aidants*", data on the typology of caregivers nationwide and the impacts of the caregiving relationship on caregivers reveal that the act of helping is not without consequences for the lives of caregivers. Many caregivers experience fatigue, exhaustion or loneliness that can lead to depression. In addition, in the majority of cases, taking charge of the illness, disability or dependence of the person being cared for leads to a loss of income, which is correlated with a change in professional life. All of these impacts, whether health, relational or financial, lead to multiple and evolving needs for caregivers (Davin et al. 2015, pp. 51–69).

Finally, a public health approach reflects the urgent need to act for caregivers. Public policies have taken up this major social and societal issue by developing a national plan for old age and loss of autonomy in 2018, in which support for caregivers is promoted. At the same time, they are prioritizing home care for people in a situation of dependence in order to rethink the care pathway and quality of life for people losing their independence. In this context, caregivers are at the heart of the mutual aid system, which is based on a balance between public intervention and family solidarity.

The *Plan Grand Âge et Autonomie* informs us that in 2018 France had more than 8 million caregivers. By 2030, there will be 1.6 million people with a loss of autonomy. In a context of an aging population where baby boomers are the ones who will need to be helped tomorrow, perpetuating the mutual aid system by improving support for caregivers is a public health issue (Bergua and Bouisson 2021).

It is from this observation that the action "By and for caregivers", carried out by DanaeCare, came about in 2019. Developed in a health democracy as an inclusive and transpathological approach, the action has mobilized associations of patients and caregivers from

Saint-Etienne and the Loire region, local authorities, health institutions and universities in order to highlight the needs of local caregivers, design adapted solutions with them and for them and document the whole system with a view to its dissemination. The aim of the whole action is to co-construct a territory that helps caregivers.

After a year of mobilization and consultation using participatory research tools, the action raised several issues related to caregiving for our territory, the main ones being the improvement of the centralization of information related to caregivers, the sensitization of health professionals and students, and the reinforcement of the territorial and administrative network.

These issues, as varied as they are, converge today in a common object, identified and identifiable by all caregivers and by the caregivers themselves: the *Escale des Aidants*, literally meaning the caregivers' port of call (I).

This whole process was fed by an action research in sociology (Chabane 2020), in which the caregiver theme constituted an object of research where societal issues and the growing capacity of caregivers to act converged (II).

By adopting an approach based on family caregivers, the entire system implemented by DanaeCare for caregivers highlights the challenges of enhancing the human relationship in healthcare through the figures and links between the caregiver and the person being cared-for. It thus questions the place of family caregivers in the healthcare system and, more generally, in our society (III).

10.2. For a territory that helps caregivers: *Escale des aidants*

The *Escale des Aidants* is the result of an unprecedented inter-associative, inter-university and inter-institutional cooperation in Saint-Étienne and the Loire region. It was designed by and for caregivers in order to co-construct a place that embodies solutions adapted to the Loire region. Eight associations, two local institutions and five faculties and schools from Saint-Etienne and the Loire region are involved in the co-construction of the *Escale des Aidants*.

In concrete terms, with an opening planned for the first quarter of 2022, the *Escale des Aidants* is a place dedicated to caregivers in the Loire region and also to a territorial strategy for caregivers. It is an innovative approach to co-constructing a territory that helps caregivers through the structuring of a caregiver network in the Loire region.

It is in this context that the "*Escale des Aidants*" resource center has emerged. Identified and identifiable by and for caregivers, it is the place where caregivers in the Loire region are welcomed, advised, informed and guided. This one-stop shop is also designed to be a place of coordination and convergence for caregivers in the Loire region in order to create an environment conducive to transpathological and multi-factorial dynamics and raise awareness of caregivers among the general public and health professionals.

In this perspective, *Escale des Aidants* acts to improve the visibility and coherence of the caregivers' pathway within the local ecosystem of caregivers.

In order to meet the time and mobility constraints of caregivers, the physical location is accompanied by a digital platform and mobile antennas. In addition to digitally enhancing the actions dedicated to caregivers implemented in our territory, the platform contains a tool to help caregivers self-identify their situation. Finally, the mobile teams will travel to the 53 municipalities of Saint-Etienne Métropole and throughout the Loire region in order to reach out to caregivers and act on their health prevention, in rural or isolated areas. By promoting the action of "going towards" the caregivers, it is a question of encouraging them to take the step of the existing devices and bring the information to them. Awareness-raising for caregivers thus takes the form of three complementary programs, aimed at meeting the concrete needs of caregivers.

From a governance point of view, *Escale des Aidants* is based on an inclusive organizational model articulated on a collaboration between an operational axis and a steering axis. On the one hand, the operational axis consists of partner associative actors and a social assistant. By acting as close as possible to the caregivers, they will animate a place open to the public, that is transpathological and participatory. On the other hand, the steering axis consists of the DanaeCare team. By anchoring itself in a collaborative approach, DanaeCare will lead the co-construction and development of *Escale des Aidants* in the service of an innovative territorial health strategy. However, the two axes are not impermeable as a monitoring committee will bring them together to follow the project's progress and deploy adjustments.

Escale des Aidants aims to respond to the needs of caregivers in the Loire Valley and propose solutions that are adapted to them. Hence, the co-construction phase has been the subject of experimentation with university partners in order to test, through multidisciplinary groups, the first responses to the needs identified.

The experimentations, launched in 2021, rely on the mobilization of students, associative actors and health professionals. The collaboration between DanaeCare, the Centre Max Weber (UJM), the EN3S and the IEP de Lyon has triggered the experimentation process on the scale of the Saint-Etienne metropolis. It resulted in the mobilization of 14 students of the master's degree students, common to the three universities, entitled "Politiques Sociales Développement Territorial (PSDT)" (Social Policies and Territorial Development) and "Politiques et innovations Sociales des Territoires (PIST)" (Social Policies and Innovations of Territories) on the experimentation field represented by DanaeCare's action "By and for caregivers". These experiments carried out in the Saint-Etienne area are part of the territorial diagnosis of caregiving and the deployment of the action in the Loire region.

Therefore, the collaboration between DanaeCare and the Health and Territory Chair of the Université Clermont Auvergne has initiated a process for the development of the spin-off strategy at the scale of the Clermont area. It took the form of a student research project (*projet mémoire recherche*, PMR) involving a group of four IAE master's students in Strategic Management at the Université Clermont Auvergne during the 2020–2021 academic year.

Consequently, the *Escale des Aidants* project, which is anchored in the "co-construction of a territory that helps caregivers" approach, is the result of inter-associative, inter-institutional and inter-university cooperation with the aim of responding coherently and appropriately to this major social and societal issue and drawing the outlines of what could be "caregiver-friendly cities".

10.3. A reflective approach in the sociology of action

The whole process related to the *Escale des Aidants* is the result of a mobilization and a consultation that was the subject of participatory workshops entitled "By and for caregivers" that brought together local caregivers for one year. These workshops were a field for sociological research (II.1). This action-research delivered its results on the issues of caregiving at the local level (II.2).

10.3.1. *Workshops by and for caregivers as a research field*

Par et pour les aidants (By and for caregivers) is a local action that brought together caregivers, patients, students, institutions (health establishments, faculties) and territorial representatives (local authorities) over a 12-month period in order to highlight issues and solutions adapted to caregivers in the care pathway and health organization. On the basis of one workshop per month, these meetings lead to the development of local solutions that can be applied in the region. The workshops, which began in January 2020, are an interesting entry point for establishing a territorial diagnosis of caregiving.

The combination of action research and health democracy makes action *By and for* caregivers a relevant field of research in the face of the intermingling of social and public health issues.

DanaeCare's monthly collective intelligence workshops were the field of study for Chabane in the framework of her master's in Social

Policies and Territorial Development. The first clear observation was the following: the theme of care is a research object at the crossroads of several policies: social, medical, public health, training, education and medicine. The recent appearance of the subject of care in the sociological field and in local social policies makes it a complex object of study to deal with, even today. Historically, and still today, it is the patients' associations that highlight the role of families in situations of illness and/or disability. We are now observing an increase in the visibility of family caregivers.

In the study of the *By and for caregivers* strategy, designed by DanaeCare, the comprehensive approach was favored by mobilizing several methods, including participant observation, processing of national and internal documentation, and the collection of caregivers' words and experiences through semi-structured interviews. These tools allowed for a concrete mobilization of health sociology. Indeed, the interest of the latter lies in the fact that the disease, and thus more broadly the caregiving, can reveal social and human relations and allow us to understand the social links that are woven around the disease and its management.

Nevertheless, while the definition of caregivers is commonly recognized, their role and their social, legal and institutional status remain unclear. Representations of "natural" assistance persist and hinder, at a certain level, a consensual social recognition of their role. So how do family caregivers organize themselves? Their *empowerment* takes various forms (discussion groups, associative groups, even pressure groups). In Saint-Etienne, family caregivers form working groups to take concrete action on local policies, while basing their expertise on their experience as caregivers.

Indeed, one of the main difficulties in studying and taking into account these helping relationships in the legal field is the following: how can we move from a social, familial and invisible role, which is confined to the "natural", to a real legal and political status? How do caregivers become beneficiaries?

The bottom-up approach chosen allows us to establish several observations. The mobilization of caregivers within local actions requires at the same time the involvement of a plurality of actors who are progressively grafted into the care pathway; the confrontation of their approaches is also essential. Thus, caregiving is never purely individual, but it is well embedded in links with others, which also allows it to be understood under the spectrum of interactionist sociology.

On the other hand, associations are often the first recourse for family caregivers in the face of local institutional disparities. The associations favored are first of all those corresponding to the pathology of the person being cared for. Thus, the strategy developed by DanaeCare, by bringing together caregivers, associations and institutions around the table, is relevant with regard to these channels where caregivers become visible on a local scale. However, before being visible by the actors of the care sector, a carer must know and dare to ask for their rights. In this field, the observation of non-use is closely linked to questions of awareness of a person's role as a carer, or not. Hence, the development of means of identification and self-identification of carers must be one of the priorities for public and social policies. Being aware of a person's role as a caregiver is inseparable from a long process of recognition by institutional, administrative, social and medical actors.

10.3.2. *Between tools and first results, what are the challenges of aid at the local level?*

A digital redefinition of workshops

The methodological choice of conducting semi-structured interviews reflects a desire to give a voice to caregivers who, according to observations during the workshops, have difficulty talking about themselves. The relevance of the interviews made sense in this comprehensive work, which revealed that this difficulty in talking about themselves is real and results from a long temporality in which the caregiver fades behind the help given to their loved one. While the discussions during the workshops took the form of an exchange of practices, the individual interviews allowed us to infiltrate the intimacy of the helping relationship and the caregiver's experience. Because of the health context, the interviews were conducted by telephone. Six caregivers gave between 45 minutes and one hour of their time to contribute to this research. One-third of the respondents represented a mother–child relationship, and one-third a sister–brother relationship. Furthermore, the average age of the respondent-caregivers was 45 years and the average age of the family caregivers was about the same (43.8 years). Among the respondents, a young caregiver (23 years old) shared his experience, thus allowing the highlighting of young caregivers, who are all the more invisible. The telephone tool made it easier for caregivers to confide in us about intimate and taboo aspects of the caregiving relationship. It is difficult to admit to the difficulty of the helping relationship when it is very prevalent. The telephone can thus reassure some people regarding the anonymity it confers. Only the voice and attentive listening are required. In fact, speaking out allows us to shed light on the experiences of these caregivers, who have not often had the opportunity to take a step back from this role, whether assumed or assigned. The consistency of the comments gives us the opportunity to question the economic, social, professional, health and institutional dimensions of the helping relationship.

While the first workshops took the form of an inventory of the situation of caregivers in the Loire region and of the existing systems, the following ones were to be devoted to a selection and a vote of potential solutions to be presented to the decision-makers. The suspension of the face-to-face workshops disrupted the progressive development of the action. The fear of losing the enthusiasm and motivation of the caregivers to take part in the action allowed us to think of other ways to conduct the workshops. The digital solution was chosen after several discussions between the DanaeCare team. Indeed, conducting an online survey seemed to be the most appropriate response to organize the vote in the shortest time possible. This survey was distributed in May–June 2020 to the network of caregivers in order to act as closely as possible to local needs. The shaping of a survey on an online platform allowed the implementation of a tool collecting the data sought. This mobilization work allowed us to broaden the representativeness of caregivers whose specificities were difficult to grasp.

This survey presents a classification of the needs identified during the first workshops and during the individual interviews. Each classification by "need" included a list of possible actions in the Saint-Etienne metropolis. To do this, it was necessary to prioritize the needs and actions, not to establish an order of preference for needs that were all essential and complementary, but to draw a roadmap or a territorial strategy that would bring visibility and effectiveness to the solutions envisaged. Each "need" corresponded to a deficiency identified in the Loire region; the "possible actions" corresponding to solutions identified for these needs. Thus, for each "need" and for each "possible solution", the respondents had to indicate a score on a scale of 0 to 10 (0 being the idea that is not or not very relevant, and 10 the idea that is very relevant). "Relevance" means any idea and action that would be the most appropriate to help aid at the local level, i.e. in the Saint-Etienne metropolis and the Loire region. Thereafter, each possible action was proposed, developed and co-constructed with institutions, territorial representatives, associations and caregivers according to the collective evaluation of its relevance resulting from the survey.

What are the responses to the needs identified? Three local issues that tend towards a local solution

During the *By and for caregivers* workshops, the relationship with the administrative and social world was mentioned several times to highlight the difficulties encountered by caregivers in the Loire Valley.

> For my brother, who has Down's syndrome, I met a social worker and she told me that your brother will be entitled to this and that, but I think that we should also and above all say what exists for us, for the caregivers. Even without saying the word caregiver, but tell them that they are not alone. They should be able to help, and guide other people who have already been through this [Anonymous interview excerpt].

The experience of the caregivers interviewed reveals the lack of territorial cohesion in the management of care and health. The aimlessness of caregivers refers to a priority given to the sick person, by the caregiver and by the social and medical actors. However, by equipping caregivers as well as possible, the repercussions on their health and well-being also benefit the entire health and administrative organization. Even if the theme of caregiving has been gaining momentum in recent years, it is important to take stock of the initiatives in order to confront them with the specific realities of the territories.

This is also in line with the difficulties that caregivers encounter when faced with the lack of networking between local authorities, which leads to a multiplication of interlocutors, constant redirections to other actors, and thus causes disruptions in the pathways of caregivers who do not find appropriate responses. The decompartmentalizing dimension of *By and for caregivers* challenges the traditional segmentation of systems and associations by pathology. Without denying the importance of having multiple structures specific to medical or social issues, the retreat of each one to its own public does not allow us to see the similarities of the experiences of caregivers, yet present in the daily life of any type of pathology. Moreover, this fragmentation creates inequalities in access to information and respite due to the lack of a sufficient territorial network.

In order to co-construct a territory that helps people to help themselves, three main issues emerge and focus our attention.

Recognizing ourselves as caregivers is not easy. However, it is much more than just helping a loved one because it involves all the dimensions of a life. However, late self-identification does not help in becoming aware of our status. Those who are able to accept it are those who have realized the magnitude of this role. The caregivers interviewed agree that there is a before-and-after phase to the caregiving relationship, but especially a turning point when they become aware of their role as caregivers.

> I used to help my husband at home with everything, I became his nurse. I had to carry him, I didn't have the right equipment. It wasn't easy and when I realized this, I was damaged. We pay the consequences in terms of

health. Now I'm the one who says it, I tell them [editor's note: the caregivers of the ASEPLS association] look at the state I'm in, I don't want you to be the same, so get help [Anonymous interview excerpt].

Invisible to professionals, caregivers are damaged. One of the challenges is to reinforce their visibility to all the actors to contribute to the concrete recognition of this role. By working to enhance the value of caregivers among the actors involved in the caregiving process, upstream, assistance in identifying caregivers should make it possible to open up a field of possibilities for the caregiver and the person being cared for in their way of fully living this relationship.

The bottom-up approach does not guarantee the representativeness of the public concerned. All the socio-cultural wealth of Saint-Etienne is not represented in these workshops. The same is true for age issues, where young caregivers who are minors or young adults are absent from the action. This second issue is particularly important when we know the heterogeneity of caregivers' profiles (the interviews conducted also contribute to this observation). We need to find other ways to identify them and raise their awareness, in particular by relying on other structures that reach a young audience. DanaeCare is currently working on a number of experiments to identify young caregivers by reaching out to them.

To date, we are faced with a lack of data on the typology of caregivers in the Loire region. The national data establishes a general quantitative picture of caregivers. At the local level, the absence of data concerning the caregivers in the territory does not facilitate a common policy of assistance to caregivers, even though we recognize the territorial disparities in access to information, access to rights and respite, depending on the pathologies of the people being cared for and the territorial initiatives. This third issue raises the need to move towards the implementation of tools to identify local caregivers, which would allow us to better understand the specificities of caregivers and implement actions adapted to their needs and situations.

The establishment of a territorial diagnosis of caregiving was necessary to prefigure the actions that could be implemented at the Loire level. These three main territorial issues lead to a local solution co-constructed with the caregivers and professionals of the territory.

To remedy territorial inconsistencies and attempt to weave a local network, work needs to be done between all the actors involved in caregiving. Among the possible ideas emanating from the *By and for caregivers* survey, the creation of a physical place specifically dedicated to caregivers is desired. Gathering all the information about the recourses available to caregivers, as well as a better knowledge of the territorial actors between them would allow a better coordination of caregivers' paths, who will then be able to identify and refer to this place as a main resource. Hence, the *Escale des Aidants* is the project that is being gradually implemented since 2020 and will be inaugurated in early 2022.

The presence of a one-stop shop in a given territory should thus promote the connection of the actors in the triptych of caregiver–patient–caregiver, while questioning the place of each in the organization of healthcare.

10.4. Conclusion: what place for caregivers in the health and social systems?

By adopting a family caregiver approach, through the prism of the human sciences and social policies, issues of value are brought to light with respect to human relations in health, through the nurse–caregiver–patient relationship. For a long time, caregivers have been considered as intruders in the world of healthcare. Without professional qualifications, these relatives intervene within the domestic space, away from the places dedicated to medical practice. Without a clearly defined status, nor a complete recognition, the legitimacy of these shadow caregivers is devalued in comparison with the professionals of this sector.

Yet, caregivers are at the heart of interrelationships in the organization of healthcare and allow for reflections around a "sanctuarization of the caregiver–patient relationship" (Simonnet and Gudefin 2019). Care is a process in which multiple stakeholders are involved – caregivers, patients, relatives, administrations, institutions, technical objects, drugs. Caregivers increasingly play a coordinating role between the various parties involved in their loved one's care. Oppositions between lay knowledge and expertise are gradually breaking down in the face of the increasing chronicity of diseases. Caregivers see the evolution of diseases on a daily basis, and their expertise is essential, especially when the people being cared for are not able to express themselves or be aware of their condition (this is the case for neurodegenerative diseases, for example). Therefore, the complementary nature of the knowledge of caregivers and social, medical and decision-making actors makes *Par et pour les aidants* relevant in its collaborative and ambitious dimension for local progress.

The participation of family caregivers in the action anchors the beginnings of caregiver awareness and empowerment in the Loire region. Caregivers, together with associative actors, embody essential resources in their quest for greater social and institutional recognition. The recognition of their experience of care, which allows for multiple questionings about social and health policies in use today, also constitutes a modality for the valorization of their role. The combination of the know-how of caregivers and professionals is crucial. A better understanding of the contribution of these two categories of actors is the basis for a progressive and long-term construction of a status for caregivers.

Finally, the importance of the role of family caregivers for the continuity and functioning of the healthcare organization has become clear in recent years. The public cause that assistance to caregivers has become attests to a full-fledged role that complements rather than replaces that of care professionals. The desire for home care coupled with public health budget cuts requires a redistribution of care practices, knowledge and skills in order to build coherent care paths. The valorization of human relations in the care pathways thus tends towards egalitarian interactions, where the reciprocal otherness between these actors constitutes the basis of the social recognition of family caregivers.

The local action of DanaeCare allows us to identify relevant lines of thought and research questions for social action and the organization of healthcare. Ongoing developments regarding traditional separations in "lay/caregiver" relationships are exposed through this field of study. Caregivers do not only provide care, and caregivers do not only cure. The intertwining of the two supports the care pathways, where a multitude of actors are involved. While the theme of caregivers is revealing of the French societal, economic and political organization, questions of recognition remain unanswered: is the lived experience sufficient to create expertise? Is the caregiver a co-caregiver? The aim here is not to answer these questions, but to stress the importance of joint work between caregivers and professionals in order to prevent situations of disruption and to co-construct a territory that supports caregivers.

Reports

DanaeCare

DanaeCare is an association under the law of 1901, founded in 2012 by André Simonnet and Julia Gudefin. Since its creation, it has conducted investigations in a dozen countries with a wide variety of health actors in medical training, organization and practice. This variety of contexts and cultures has highlighted that the human relationship in health, and in particular the nurse/patient/caregiver relationship, is the fertile ground for fostering a sustainable health ecosystem for nurses, patients, caregivers and the health organization. Today, changes in human relationships in healthcare are impacting the organization and care pathway at different levels and degrees. Hence, DanaeCare aims to put the human relationship back at the heart of care by perceiving it as the new indicator of tomorrow's medicine.

10.5. References

Bergua, V. and Bouisson, J. (eds) (2021). *Pour aider les aidants, osons l'aidance*. Editions In Press, Paris.

Chabane, M. (2020). Valorisation du rôle et du statut des proches aidants. L'action locale de DanaeCare pour une catégorie incertaine de l'action publique. Thesis, Université Jean Monnet, Saint-Étienne.

Davin, B., Paraponaris, A., Protiere, C. (2015). Pas de prix mais un coût ? Évaluation contingente de l'aide informelle apportée aux personnes âgées en perte d'autonomie. *Économie et Statistique*, 475–476, 51–69.

Rossinot, H. (2019). *Aidants, ces invisibles*. Editions de l'Observatoire, Paris.

Simonnet, A. and Gudefin, J. (2019). La relation soignant-patient, le nouvel indicateur de la médecine de demain ? *Techniques hospitalières*, 774, 57–60.

List of Authors

Abdelhadi BELLACHHAB
PREFICS
Université de Nantes
France

Ibtissem BEN DRIDI
École des Hautes Études en
Santé Publique (EHESP)
Rennes and Arènes Laboratory
(UMR CNRS 6051)
Rennes
France

Aicha BENABED
Department of Sociology and
Anthropology
Faculty of Social Sciences
University of Oran 2
and
Health and Social Sciences
Research Unit (GRAS)
University of Oran 2
Bir El Djir
Algeria

Maya CHABANE
DanaeCare
Saint-Étienne
France

Christelle CHAUZAL-LARGUIER
Management Sciences
Communication and Societies
Laboratory
Université Clermont Auvergne
Clermont-Ferrand
France

Emna CHERIF
CleRMa
Université Clermont Auvergne
Clermont-Ferrand
France

Laurence CORROY
Centre de Recherche sur les
médiations (CREM)
Université de Lorraine
Nancy
France

Ambre DAVAT
TIMC/GRESEC Laboratories
Universitaire Grenoble Alpes
France

Aurélia DUMAS
Information and
Communication Sciences (ICS)
Laboratoire Communication
et Sociétés
Université Clermont Auvergne
Clermont-Ferrand
France

Olga GALATANU
PREFICS
Université de Nantes
France

Nathalie GARRIC
PREFICS
Université de Nantes
France

Julia GUDEFIN
DanaeCare
Saint-Étienne
France

Fabienne MARTIN-JUCHAT
GRESEC Laboratory
Universitaire Grenoble Alpes
France

Alexis MEYER
Université Clermont Auve
Clermont-Ferrand
France

Julie PAVILLET
Centre Hospitalier
Universitaire Grenoble Al
France

Frédéric PUGNIÈRE-SAAVI
PREFICS
Université Bretagne Sud
Lorient
France

Valérie ROCHAIX
Laboratoire Ligérien de
Linguistique (LLL)
CNRS 7270
Université de Tours
France

Emilie ROCHE
Centre de recherche sur le
liens sociaux (CERLIS)
Université Sorbonne Nou
Paris
France

Corinne ROCHETTE
CleRMa
Health and Territories Cha
Université Clermont Auve
Clermont-Ferrand
France

André SIMONNET
DanaeCare
Saint-Étienne
France

Anne VEGA
Sophiapol
Université de Nanterre
and
CENS
Université de Nantes
France

Index

Other titles from

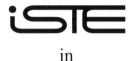

in

Health Engineering and Society

2023

Beyala Laure
Digital Therapy: The New Age of Healthcare
(Technological Prospects and Social Applications Set – Volume 6)

2022

Assailly Jean-Pascal
Child Psychology: Developments in Knowledge and Theoretical Models
(Health and Patients Set – Volume 3)

Chaabane Sondès, Cousein Etienne, Wieser Philippe
Healthcare Systems: Challenges and Opportunities

Paganelli Céline, Clavier Viviane
Information Practices and Knowledge in Health
(Health and Patients Set – Volume 5)

Salgues Bruno, Barnouin Jacques
The Covid-19 Crisis: From a Question of an Epidemic to a Societal
Questioning
(Health and Patients Set – Volume 4)

2021

BÉRANGER Jérôme
Societal Responsibility of Artificial Intelligence: Towards an Ethical and Eco-responsible AI
(Technological Prospects and Social Applications Set – Volume 4)

CORDELIER Benoit, GALIBERT Olivier
Digital Health Communications
(Technological Prospects and Social Applications Set – Volume 5)

NADOT Michel
Discipline of Nursing: Three-time Knowledge

2020

BARBET Jacques, FOUCQUIER Adrien, THOMAS Yves
Therapeutic Progress in Oncology: Towards a Revolution in Cancer Therapy?
(Health and Patients Set – Volume 2)

MORILLON Laurent, CLAVIER Viviane
Health Research Practices in a Digital Context
(Health Information Set – Volume 4)

PAILLIART Isabelle
New Territories in Health
(Health Information Set – Volume 3)

2019

CLAVIER Viviane, DE OLIVEIRA Jean-Philippe
Food and Health: Actor Strategies in Information and Communication
(Health Information Set – Volume 2)

PIZON Frank
Health Education and Prevention
(Health and Patients Set – Volume 1)

2018

HUARD Pierre
The Management of Chronic Diseases: Organizational Innovation and Efficiency

PAGANELLI Céline
Confidence and Legitimacy in Health Information and Communication (Health Information Set – Volume 1)

2017

PICARD Robert
Co-design in Living Labs for Healthcare and Independent Living: Concepts, Methods and Tools

2015

BÉRANGER Jérôme
Medical Information Systems Ethics